RUN MUMMY RUN

RUN MUMMY RUN

Summersdale Publishers Ltd
46 West Street
Chichester
West Sussex
PO19 1RP
UK

www.summersdale.com

Printed and bound by CPI Group (UK) Ltd, Croydon, CR0 4YY

ISBN: 978-1-78685-237-3

Substantial discounts on bulk quantities of Summersdale books are available to corporations, professional associations and other organisations. For details contact general enquiries: telephone: +44 (0) 1243 771107 or email: enquiries@summersdale.com.

Disclaimer
Neither the authors nor the publisher can be held responsible for any injury, loss or claim arising out of the use, or misuse, of the suggestions made herein.

Leanne Davies and
Lucy Waterlow

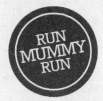

RUN MUMMY RUN

Inspiring Women
to Be Fit,
Healthy and Happy

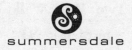

summersdale

CONTENTS

INTRODUCTION

Hello and welcome to the Run Mummy Run book! I'm Leanne, or Mummy to some, and I am the founder of Run Mummy Run, an online running community that inspires and supports women to be fit, happy and healthy. I'm not an elite athlete or running coach – I'm just a mum who loves to run for all the good it brings, and I'm passionate about helping other women do the same.

You might already know about the Run Mummy Run community, but if you don't, let me tell you a little about how it started and how it can help you. It all began when I created a Facebook group in 2012 so a handful of friends and I could motivate one another to run, as I was struggling to fit in any exercise after becoming a mum of two. I never imagined that the group would become a nationwide network of thousands of like-minded women, all supporting and encouraging one another to run no matter their speed or ability.

I ran a lot before becoming a mum, taking part in the odd half marathon and doing a full one in 2008. Back then, I had the freedom to run whenever I wanted, I could enter races as and when I pleased, and I had friends to run with who could do the same. This all changed when I had children. I tried to keep the momentum going but it became so much harder to get out for a run as the responsibility of looking after two little boys overtook the ease of popping my trainers on. I'd often arrange to meet a friend for a run only to have to pull out at the last minute if my husband was late home from work or I had to look after a poorly little one. I would have loved to have joined a local running club but, as no week was ever the same, I couldn't commit to regularly making their evening sessions. Whenever my husband could hold the fort and I could get out the door, it would often be late on cold, dark nights when I would pound the pavements alone. I missed having company and the support of other runners to chat to about my running highs and lows. Running didn't seem so fun anymore.

In December 2012, when I finally met one of my good running pals, Wendy, for a run, I told her about my frustrations and decided it was time I did something about it. What did I need? A network of like-minded women who shared my love of running and wanted to talk about it. On my return home from our run I sat in my kitchen, had a coffee and set up a closed Facebook group, inviting Wendy and one other female friend to join. It just seemed like an easier way to arrange to meet up and have a group chat rather than sending multiple text messages. As well as arranging runs, we motivated and encouraged one another to get out the door, especially on the days when we had no choice but to go alone and staying inside in the warm felt more appealing. We also shared our kit recommendations, funny experiences and the running knowledge we were gaining via trial and error.

Soon, more friends in the area wanted to join, and then friends of friends, until we had 30 members. Brilliant, I thought, job done. Then every day I kept getting more and more requests from women who wanted to join. They were no longer from my local area but from all across the UK. The group steadily grew in popularity; before I knew it we had 1,000 members, then 5,000 and now, at the time of writing, over 50,000. It has grown beyond just me and my love of running to a leading national network for female runners, bringing together tens of thousands of women with a shared passion for running and a penchant for colourful compression socks. We've gone on to be named *Women's Running* magazine's Influencer of the Year, won gold three times at The Running Awards and have been invited to become official supporters of Cancer Research UK's Race For Life series and Sport England's This Girl Can campaign.

What makes the group so special is the people in it, as they give such amazing support and encouragement to one another. The positivity is infectious. No one is ever judged or criticised. It remains a closed group so women can share personal or sensitive matters related to running in a safe and understanding environment. We actively promote kindness and inclusivity. All you need is a friendly smile and a love of running to be in the club. Despite the name of the group, you don't even have to be a mum. All women are welcome, whether they have children or not.

Our aim is to encourage and inspire all women to take up running and enjoy their journey. We want to be there to help them through the tough times, share their milestones and celebrate their achievements. We want to provide a safe, secure environment where women can talk openly about every aspect of running and know they'll be met with kindness, respect and love. We're passionate about encouraging the next generation to be active, and we believe that by supporting women in their running journeys they become role-models for their children, thereby inspiring them and promoting self-belief.

We've discovered that strangers quickly become friends via the group. We offer opportunities to make our community more than just a virtual one by organising formal RMR meet-ups at races, official group runs in scenic locations and motivational talks with experts. Members can also organise among themselves to meet up at races or to go on training runs.

As many members started asking where they could find fashionable and functional sports gear, we also launched our own online branded merchandise store, which sells running clothing and accessories. We want to provide high quality running kit that is designed for female runners, by female runners, so we take our time thoroughly researching every product we sell. We want our members to feel proud to identify themselves as part of the RMR tribe.

With this book, we hope to give you a taste of the RMR community and help you get active. The book covers the most common topics raised in the group from how to get started with a Couch To 5k plan to how to pluck up the courage to enter a race. There's also advice on avoiding injury, the best foods for runners and how to fit running in around work and family life, plus training plans to help you along the way.

Many women love RMR because it's a place where they can ask questions they might be too embarrassed to ask anywhere else – how to run when you're on your period, or how to avoid an uncomfortable call of nature on a long training run – so there's a chapter bringing together some of these common problems too.

If you're new to running, there may be lots of terms you are unfamiliar with. You might not know what your IT band is, let alone how it can affect your running, be bewildered by the comic-sounding fartlek run, or wonder if you have to be a naturist to achieve a running 'streak'. So there's a glossary at the back to help you understand a runner's lingo. There're also a few terms in there that have become synonymous for RMR members over the years, such as 'Jeffing' and 'cockwombles', so check out the glossary for clarification if you're ever confused by what we're talking about!

Hopefully this book will inspire you to start, restart or keep running. If you live in the UK and you're not already a member of our Facebook group then do come and join us to share your journey and get lots of support. The community has definitely proved to be the answer I was looking for; not only has it given me the motivation and encouragement I needed to get out there and run, I have also been lucky enough to make many friends and meet some truly inspirational women along the way. I'm proud of how Run Mummy Run has become such a kind, friendly and supportive place for women to get active and follow their dreams. It's changed my life for the better and I hope it can do the same for you.

Enjoy reading, and happy running!

Leanne

CHAPTER ONE:
BABY STEPS

REASONS TO RUN – HEALTH AND HAPPINESS
(AND EATING CAKE!)

The one question an inquisitive toddler is guaranteed to ask if they see you running past them on the street or in the park is: 'Why is that lady running, Mummy?' It would actually take a mum (or dad) all day to explain why, as there are so many reasons why we do it.

Let's start with the physical benefits – running can keep your heart healthy, strengthen your bones, muscles and tendons and reduce your risk of developing a serious illness like cancer. So it is perhaps no surprise that numerous studies have found that runners live longer than inactive people.

Running will also make you feel stronger and more toned, which will boost your body-confidence and self-esteem. As running raises the heart rate and burns calories – around 100 per mile on average – it will help you maintain a healthy weight while still allowing you to treat yourself occasionally with cake and chocolate. That's a big plus for us!

There's nothing like a good run in the fresh air to clear your head and make you feel on top of the world, and that's because running releases endorphins. These are the feel-good hormones that can reduce symptoms of depression, which is why running is also great for your mental health. Exercise is also a stress-reliever, so you will often find a problem that was troubling you before a run seems so much more manageable once you've returned feeling invigorated.

For mums, running is a fantastic form of exercise because you can fit it in as and when you can around your children. You can even take them with you, either by using a running buggy or by doing a fun run together (although some of our members will tell you they would rather leave the kids behind when they run as it's their time to relax and get away from it all for half an hour!).

Many women love to run because it's such a sociable activity. You can go with friends and put the world to rights in the process, and meet many new people by joining a running group or club. It might not be a traditional team sport, but you can still team up with your running buddies to face a race together.

Racing is another reason why many love to run. It allows them to come together with others who share their passion in an exciting atmosphere. Finishing a race can give you a real sense of achievement and can drive you to want to race again and go further or faster next time.

Understanding why you run is important as it will help you stay motivated on the days when you can't face getting up and going out, or if you find yourself struggling to keep going when you do. Here is some motivation from RMR members who told us why they run...

'I run for my health, to inspire my little boys and to spark new friendships.'
Leanne Davies

'I run to explore, to compete, to socialise – and so I can eat cake!'
Lucy Waterlow

'I started running in my forties – I knew I couldn't stop middle age but I could stop myself becoming more sluggish and unfit.'
Fiona Godden

'I run because my son can't. I'm a single mum to a profoundly disabled, gorgeous little boy who was diagnosed with a life-limiting condition. Running helps me zone out and clear my mind.'
Tracie Kirby

'I run to escape! It's my "me" time away from three young children. Being a stay-at-home mum is hard work and running is my mental and physical stress release.'
Hayley Milam

'I started to run to lose weight but discovered so much more. It has given me a newfound confidence in myself and I've made some amazing friends.'
Hannah Jones

'I was dared to run a marathon. Along the way I found out that I really enjoy getting away from the kids' constant squabbles and "mum mum mum".'
Elizabeth Clair Ayres

'I run so I can eat chocolate, for head-space and to set a healthy example for my little girl.'
Elaine Diffenthal

'I run because it's the only time I get to be me! Not the nurse, the carer, the mum. Just me. It's my therapy. I put the world to rights in my head and return calmer. Running is escapism in its simplest form.'
Nicola Carter

'I run because I was told I couldn't. I was always too fat, thin, ill, busy etc. I hope to be a role-model to my kids as I overcame my demons and gave two fingers to the doubters who said I couldn't.'

Emma Thompson

'I started running to lose weight and get fit because I was worried about getting ill and not being there for my children. Now I run to feel strong and healthy, to have time to myself and to see beautiful places.'

Gillian Ross

'I started running to help with postnatal depression, asthma and psoriatic arthritis. Now my asthma is stable, I take no pain medication or antidepressants and I can keep up with four boys!'

Louise Leeder

'Running helps me deal with the stress and anxiety I have due to my son's (at times) challenging behaviour as a result of his Autism Spectrum Disorder. It helps keep me sane and healthy.'

Rebecca Measures Amos

'I run for peace of mind and to keep myself fit for my children and grandchildren.'
Suzanne L'oreal Fennell

'I run for head-space and to be the best mum I can be.'
Catherine Mulrenan

'I run to be me, to be free and to feel like I'm five years old again without a care in the world.'
Katie Griffiths

'I run because it makes me feel strong. It makes me focus on what my body can do, not what it looks like.'
Paula Sheridan

'It's exercise that is relatively cheap that you can do straight out of your front door.'
Rachel Finsbury

'I run to fundraise for my son who was two when he died from his first asthma attack. I have a place in the London Marathon in 2018. We hope to get to a total of one hundred thousand pounds.'
Gemma Brown

'I run to help with my anxiety and depression – there's nothing like an endorphin boost!'
Nicola Wood

'I was the girl who never got picked for sports but I started running when my dad was diagnosed with terminal cancer. When he became really ill, running kept me sane and really helped me to cope with stress and grief.'
Jenine Cooper

'As a cancer survivor, I run looking for the next goal to raise money and awareness, to better myself and hopefully inspire others too.'
Louise Vernon

'I have chronic lung disease so I run because I can. One day I'll be sat in a chair fighting for breath and unable to run again, so I want to live my life now, not wait for that chair to catch up with me.'
Rachael Oldfield

'I had depression on and off for a number of years. If I have a down day, I go for a run. I look forward to running, exploring new places and just getting out there to get moving. Running has changed my life for the better.'

Sarah Beeley

'Running has given me such a sense of achievement in myself and pride that I can, and will, do whatever I put my mind to.'

Vicki White Webb

SHE BELIEVED SHE COULD, SO SHE DID: OVERCOMING FEAR OF EXERCISE

It might be the case that you know all the reasons why you *should* be running to improve your health and happiness and you would love to be able to do it – but you just don't think you can. Research carried out by Sport England in 2014 found that 75 per cent of women in England aged 14–40 wanted to exercise more but were put off by fears of being judged about their fitness and body shape. When it comes to running, many are reluctant to be seen getting red-faced and sweaty, or with their 'wobbly bits' jiggling, as they believe running is only for the super slim and speedy. Fortunately, the tide has started to turn thanks to Sport England's This Girl Can campaign, which has shown that women of all shapes and sizes can exercise. This is something we fully believe at RMR too. It doesn't matter what you look like or whether you are tall, short, large or small. There is no ideal body shape to be a runner.

Another barrier for many women is a belief they just can't run. This may be down to bad past experiences of hating PE at school or the old cliché of struggling to run for a bus. While there are rare health complications that prevent some from running, for the majority of women it's not their body holding them back but their mindset. You need to have self-belief and to stop telling yourself you can't do it. It may feel hard at first as it can take a few weeks to build up fitness but you can be a runner, even if you haven't attempted running since childhood. Being a runner doesn't mean you have to be super-fast or run a long distance either – it's just about getting out and getting fit for all the benefits it brings. A favourite slogan at RMR is: 'she believed she could, so she did.' Keep it in mind next time you have any negative thoughts preventing you from going for your first run, entering a race or joining a running group. You can do it!

One of our members who sums up this philosophy is Sara Spells, 44, who has gone on to become an ultrarunner after once believing she couldn't even run a mile. She said: 'I used to be overweight and believed I wasn't built for running. At school, I would often fake an ankle injury to get out of doing PE. In my forties, I finally plucked up the courage to do a Couch To 5k course at my local gym as I was told losing weight could help me conceive. What a life-changer it has been! I have progressed beyond my wildest expectations.

I have lost six stone, had three children and finished an ultramarathon. Running has given me confidence, a belief in myself that anything is possible and lots of friends. It also helped me deal with my grief after suffering a number of miscarriages, including the loss of my third daughter, Hope, when I was twenty-three weeks pregnant. I would say to anyone who thinks they can't be a runner – always believe in yourself. So what if sometimes you have to walk, or if you're slower than others? You're still doing it.'

BE FEARLESS BUT STAY SAFE

It's wonderful to feel empowered and fearless through running, but don't forget to stay safe and look out for one another.

▶ **Safety in numbers:** Running with someone else is not only more fun, it's also safer. When possible, arrange to run with a friend or join a local running group so you're not going alone. If you are an absolute beginner, do check a running group or club is suitable for your level of fitness first. It doesn't happen very often, but some RMR members have reported being left behind on a run after going to a club for the first time because they couldn't keep up with the pace. Not only has this left them lost or vulnerable, they've also found it disheartening. However, don't let this put you off joining a club as many will offer training suitable for all abilities – they are not only the preserve of the super fit. Just check in advance that they can cater for beginners. If they don't, there's bound to be another group in your area that does, such as one running a Couch To 5k course. Try searching the England Athletics directory at www.runtogether.co.uk/groups/, and of course you can ask for recommendations in your area via the RMR page. It can be intimidating going to a club for the first time, especially if you feel everyone else is fitter than you, but it's worth plucking up the courage as there are so many benefits beyond the safety-in-numbers aspect. RMR members who have joined running clubs say they have made many friends and it has helped their confidence and fitness soar.

Another way to easily run with others if you don't have anyone you can meet with regularly is to join in a parkrun every Saturday at 9 a.m. These are free, timed 5k runs (not races) in parks across the UK and other parts of the world, including Australia and Denmark. All abilities are welcome; you can even walk the whole way if you can't run (read more about parkrun in chapter five, page 145).

▶ **Plan and share your route:** It isn't always possible or convenient to meet someone for every run, so if you are going alone tell someone your intended route and how long you expect to be gone. Take your mobile phone so you are able to make contact in case of emergency. There are some apps you can download that enable a friend or partner to track you during a run, so while they might not be physically beside you they can still check that you are okay. One example is Strava, which has a 'beacon' feature that alerts three friends to a run you are doing and will tell them if you stop for a long period of time. It's worth using technology like this if you have to do long training runs alone that take you far from home.

If you are running by yourself, avoid secluded, rarely-trodden paths. Some women deliberately run on isolated routes at quiet hours of the day to avoid being seen exercising in public. If this is you then please don't let being self-conscious go ahead of being sensible, it really isn't worth the risk. Although it is rare to be attacked while on a run, sadly it can happen, so don't put yourself in any situations where you will be vulnerable.

▶**Listen up:** While it's fine to have entertainment on the run to help you pass the time, such as music, an audiobook or a podcast, be careful that you don't get too lost in your own thoughts. Don't run in headphones that have been designed to cut out background noise and don't have the volume cranked up too high – you still need to be able to hear what else is going on around you, from passing traffic to someone approaching from behind. When racing, you have to be able to hear any instructions from marshals, so for this reason some road races now ban participants from wearing headphones.

▶**Be safe, be seen:** If you're running before sunrise, at twilight or after dark then high visibility clothing is essential. Fluorescent colours work well for the dawn and twilight hours but at night you need to wear something reflective that will bounce the light from a car's headlights off you so you can be seen by the driver. There are also many small, flashing lights now on sale that you can wear or clip onto your clothing to light yourself like a Christmas tree. Another option is to wear a head torch. This will allow you both to be seen by others and to light your path where streetlights are unavailable or inadequate.

▶ **Carry ID:** These events are rare, but if you are involved in an accident or have a sudden health problem that renders you speechless when out running, carrying ID will let paramedics know who you are and enable them to contact your next of kin quickly. If you're running with your mobile, add your ICE (in case of emergency) details to your contacts. Customised ICE identity bracelets are also available to buy which you can wear when running. These bracelets list emergency contact details, as well as potentially life-saving information such as any medications you are taking or allergies you suffer from.

When racing, organisers will often ask you to write this information on the back of your race number. Get into the habit of filling it in as one of your pre-race rituals. It's unlikely you will get into difficulties but it's always better to be safe than sorry.

HOW TO FIT RUNNING INTO YOUR BUSY LIFE AND STAY SANE

Another barrier to exercise for many women is just finding the time. Running is a 'vigorous aerobic activity' according to the NHS, and it's recommended that adults do 75 minutes of this kind of exercise every week in order to stay healthy. That means running for 25 minutes three times a week. To some it may not sound like a lot, but to mums who barely even have a minute to go to the toilet, it can seem absurd. These are just the minimal recommended running times to stay healthy too. If your goal is to run a long distance race, like a half marathon or marathon, you'll have to spend more than 75 minutes training each week. So how are you going to do it? You might feel the odds are stacked against you if you're juggling full or part-time work with motherhood, or you're a single parent. But don't give up hope. Thousands of RMR members before you have also wondered how on earth they can squeeze any exercise into their busy lives and they have managed to find a way. Here we have brought together some of their top tips to help you.

▶**Be an early bird:** Set your alarm, throw on your trainers and catch the sunrise while the rest of the world (and hopefully your children) still slumber. Many RMR members say rising and running sets them up for the day ahead and gives them a chance to enjoy some peace and quiet before the chaos that may follow. Some even admit to sleeping in their running gear to help them get up and out before their children wake up! If your little ones are early risers it might mean you have to run as early as 4 or 5 a.m., but RMR members who do this regularly say it is not as hideous as you might think. One of them, Tinu Ogundari says: 'I run at four thirty in the morning before I get the children ready for school. I live in London and at that time it is so peaceful and quiet, unlike in the evening when it's noisy and there are too many obstacles which mean I can't concentrate on the running. Early-morning runs kickstart your day and make you feel alive and ready to do anything you want to achieve.'

Lorna Davis agrees. She says: 'I'm an early-morning runner as my husband's work means I can never depend on what time he'll be home in the evening, plus I work nights. It's tough in the winter when mornings are dark, but I love the quietness and lack of people; I can just get my head down and put in the miles. It gives me loads more energy for the day ahead too.'

Emma Louise adds: 'I'm an early-morning runner. I started so I couldn't make excuses about being too tired after work. Now I do it because I love the solitude and the quiet!'

▶ **Find a running buddy-babysitter:** Finding childcare so you can run can be tricky, especially if you are a single parent, have a partner who works long hours or don't have any other relatives living locally to lend a hand. But what you can be sure of is that you're not the only mum in this situation, so what you need to do is join forces! Find another mum with similar childcare issues in your area and then offer to take it in turns to babysit for one another while the other goes for a run. You could do this as a relay – going one after the other on the same day – or arrange to take it in turns with one person running while the other babysits one day, and swapping roles another day. This running-childcare trade also gives you the chance to get out and meet another mum, as you can share a cuppa and a chat together after your run while the kids play – it's win-win!

▶ **Run with a buggy:** When your baby is old enough, you could consider taking them running with you in a buggy. Unfortunately it can't be just any buggy though – it must be one specially adapted for running which has large inflatable wheels and a fixed front wheel to ensure a smooth and safe ride for your precious cargo. Before using a running buggy, make sure you double check the manufacturer's instructions to ensure your child is old enough to ride in it. For some they must be six months, while for others they must be from eight to nine months onwards. Do not run with a child in the running buggy before they reach the recommended age for the product. Most manufacturers advise that babies should have the strength to hold their own head up before they go in a running buggy, so also be mindful of your child's individual development, as all babies progress at different rates.

To make it easier for you to run with, running buggies have adjustable handlebars and rear wheels that are set widely to give more room at your feet – this allows you to run without shortening your stride. If you have a wide path to run along, you can also run alongside the buggy, holding one corner of it to steer. The buggies have a wrist strap to ensure it can't slip from your grasp, a handbrake to control your speed (especially important when running downhill) and, of course, a safety harness to keep your little one firmly strapped in.

We are lucky to have many running buggy pros in the RMR community and one of them is Wendy Rumble, founder of RunningBuggies.com. When running with a buggy, she recommends pushing it with one arm and swinging the other, and alternating each arm over time (making sure you change over the wrist strap when you do this). She also advises runners not to lean on the handlebars, as this could cause tension in your back. She adds: 'Ensure your elbows are at ninety degrees by setting the handlebars at the right height which again helps make sure you are upright. Do not change your stride and avoid the temptation to point your toes out. Instead, keep them facing forward – a running buggy should allow for this so you still have space to run.'

To prepare your baby for the ride, Rumble says: 'Build up the distances gradually so that your baby gets used to it. Remember to pack your rain cover as it also comes in handy when it's windy for some shelter. Take a few bits with you in the various pockets in the buggy; a change roll with wipes and a nappy, kids' snacks, drinks for you both and some toys. But tie them on! When it comes to drinks and snacks, make sure they are spill proof so your child doesn't get damp and cold if they spill something on themselves.'

If you fear your child won't want to sit still long enough for you to run, time it with their nap so they can snooze while you pursue your running dreams!

This can be an expensive option, as running buggies cost between £100 and £300, but you could see it as money well spent if it gets you and your child out of the house. You'll be investing in your own physical and mental health and saving on potential childcare fees by taking your child with you. However, if you are looking to be economical, opt for a model that you could use as a buggy for your other daily activities as well so you don't need to buy more than one. You could also look for a second-hand model.

▶**Bring the older ones along:** Running is a wonderful and inexpensive way to keep active as a family, so if you have kiddies that will no longer fit in a buggy, turn your run into a fun activity that they can join in with. Older children can run with you and younger ones could accompany you riding a bike or a scooter. Alternatively, your partner could ride their bike with your child in a seat – they will be perfectly placed to hold onto your water bottle and pass it to you when you need it! You could also join in a 5k parkrun or 2k junior parkrun (read more on parkrun in chapter five) together at weekends, and look for other local fun runs that you can all participate in as a family. Around Christmas, there are often Santa fun runs that kids love as they can dress up in festive attire.

▶**Gym childcare:** Some gyms offer crèche facilities bookable by the hour. Affordability is always a factor but, if feasible, it's a great option for grabbing that well-deserved hour just for you.

▶**Run to or from work, or even in your lunch hour:** Providing you live within a reasonable distance and there are shower facilities at your workplace, a run-commute is ideal for fitting in your exercise without impacting on personal or family time. All you will need is a running rucksack to enable you to run comfortably with the essentials. Coordinating what you need to pack is important, but once you've done it a few times you'll be a pro! You could also plan to leave some items (such as smart shoes) at your workplace so you aren't carrying as much.

Another option if your commute is too far to run is to go in your lunch hour and eat at your desk when you return. It will be a much better afternoon pick-me-up than another coffee.

A run-commute will save you money on transport and you'll feel pretty fabulous sitting at your desk knowing your run is done for the day. Or, if you run home, you'll know that as soon as you get in the door the rest of the evening is yours to relax in. Bliss.

▶ **Why drive when you can run?** When it comes to swapping driving and public transport for trainers, you don't have to stop at your commute. Are there other journeys in your everyday life that you could run? Having a running buggy will help if you have to take the children as you could, for example, run them to doctors' appointments and play groups. If you're planning to go somewhere as a family, could you run home while your partner drives the children back? It will require forward planning but you might find it surprisingly easy to fit in a run when you switch four wheels for your two feet.

▶ **Buy a treadmill:** If you have the space in your home for a treadmill, you can run while your children are sleeping.

It might not be as much fun or as invigorating as running outdoors but it will still allow you to keep fit – and might be preferable on evenings when it's dark, cold and pouring with rain! This is an expensive option, but you could try to find one second-hand to keep the cost down.

▶**Schedule your runs:** Plan ahead to ensure you make time for running. If you keep a diary, write in your runs around everything else you have planned. If you see it written into your schedule, you will be more likely to go. Planning to go to a running club session will also help as you can factor their meeting time into your day.

However you decide to fit your running in, make sure you don't stress over it. Our lives are manic enough without adding more worries. Once you have found a way to run, try to stay in the same routine for a few weeks so it becomes a habit. Choose a method that fits comfortably with your life and always remember: ten minutes is better than no minutes at all.

RMR STORIES

'Running feels part of me now': RMR's Michelle Foreman, 40, a wife, mother-of-three and running coach from Westgate-on-Sea, Kent, who works as a vulnerable persons' officer for the fire service (after 15 years as a fire fighter) reveals why she runs and how she fits it into her jam-packed schedule.

It's 5 a.m. and I'm creeping around the house pulling on my kit before quietly closing the front door and heading out for an early-morning run.

Training at the crack of dawn is one of the ways I manage to fit in exercise so it doesn't impact on my family time. I can be back from my run before my husband, two sons aged 12 and 10 and daughter, seven, have gotten out of bed. Then I have the rest of the day to devote to them.

I usually run about 20 miles a week, rising to 30–40 when I'm marathon training. I started young as my father was athletic, so I grew up surrounded by sport. I ran for the school cross country team and played for a football club.

Running feels part of me now. I don't feel like me unless I am training or have something to aim for. However, now I'm a wife and mother of three and working for the fire service, fitting in training is a lot harder than it used to be.

To make it work, as well as going out early, I also join in my local parkrun with my husky dog most Saturday mornings.

Being part of a running club has also made a huge difference to my training and motivation. I have become an England Athletics qualified coach so I train juniors for a club on Monday evenings, and lead group runs for adults at my running club on Wednesday evenings and Sunday mornings.

I'd recommend joining a club to everyone as it's sociable and the regular sessions will become a routine part of your life. I have made some of my best friends through my current club, Alfie's Striders (www.alfiestrust.com), named after a local boy who had cancer and sadly died at the age of two. His parents set up a charity to fund a ward at Great Ormond Street Hospital and our running club fundraises for them.

It isn't the first club I have been part of but it is the one that's my perfect fit. So I would say to people, if at first you don't find a club that suits you, then go along to another, and don't give up.

My husband works in Formula One so he's often away travelling the world, which can curtail my training. My 76-year-old mother babysits on some evenings when he's away so I can still make club nights. To single parents, I would advise trying to get a family member to help you out regularly so you can still train. Or you could get a second-hand treadmill so you can run at home. I have one and I make training on it more interesting by mixing up what I do. Some days I might do a ten-minute HIIT session, others a 15-minute incline walk. If you can position it in front of a TV, it also helps pass the time!

Again, I would advise parents who want to run to join a club. You might be able to take your children with you, as some allow kids to join in on scooters and in running buggies. Or, if they are old enough, they could join in a junior session while you do your own training.

If you are in a relationship, try to get your partner to support your training. My husband isn't a runner so I adapt my running so it doesn't encroach on family life too much, as otherwise it can cause resentment. That's why I tend to go early in the mornings or in the evenings when the children have gone to bed.

If your partner is a runner and you have children, you can take it in turns to go, or even do an interval session where one of you does a lap of the block while the other waits doing star jumps with the children, and then you keep swapping places. There are lots of ways to make it work.

I never take being able to run for granted, as I suffer from M.E. When my children were young it became so bad I wasn't able to run for three years. I then had to build my training back up gradually. I still get occasional relapses but it only stops me running now for a couple of weeks at a time.

I also stay motivated by continually setting myself race targets. This year, I ran the Brighton Marathon and then the London Marathon two weeks later. It took a lot out of me but I loved the experiences and raised money with my fellow Alfie's Striders in the process.

I know it can be tiring to combine training with a job and/or motherhood but I always say to the women I coach, 'If you don't feel like it, just put your shoes on and do a mile. I can guarantee once you're out, you'll feel like your legs have another mile in them.'

My other tops tips are to do a Couch To 5k plan if you are just starting out. Take it slowly when you begin to run to avoid getting injured. Get a good pair of trainers and, just as importantly, a decent sports bra.

I also advocate strength training, especially exercises to 'fire up' the glutes, such as squats and lunges (see page 82 for more on this). It will aid your running form and prevent injury. You don't have to join a gym as you can do these exercises at home.

And, of course, I highly recommend joining RMR. I was told about the group by a friend. As soon as I was added, I spent ages scrolling through all the posts. I loved it – the motivation and seeing how everyone there is so caring. It's full of women who are beautiful inside and out.

Life is short, so I believe you have to grasp it with both hands and keep challenging yourself. There's such a beautiful world out there and running can help you explore it.

ALL THE GEAR, NO IDEA? WHAT YOU ACTUALLY NEED, INDULGENCES YOU COULD RUN WITHOUT (BUT SHOULD GET ANYWAY) AND WHAT YOU CAN DEFINITELY DITCH

Thanks to running becoming more popular, particularly with women, there's now a multitude of activewear in the shops. The choice can be overwhelming so the RMR page is often full of confused members asking for recommendations. Picking the right kit can be crucial in ensuring you have a comfortable, enjoyable run so it's best to go with brands and products specifically designed with runners in mind. And it is possible to get kit that is fashionable as well as functional! As we've said before, appearances don't matter, but if you are self-conscious about running you'll feel so much better if you go in gear that is flattering and makes you feel good.

Running is said to be a cheap sport to take up but with the array of clothing, gadgets and accessories available you could soon find you max out your credit card once you've been bitten by the running bug! So, if you're on a budget, what do you actually need and what should you avoid wasting your money on?

THE ESSENTIALS

▶**Trainers:** Finding the right running shoe for you is an absolute must to avoid injury and ensure you have happy feet. Some can be pricey but even budget supermarkets sell running trainers nowadays, so you don't have to spend a fortune. Getting the right fit and feel for you is more important than how much you spend. Just ensure they are trainers that have been specifically designed for running.

To avoid rubbing blisters they shouldn't be too tight, particularly around the toes and heel; many find going half a size or even a whole size up from what they would usually wear is best. If you go up a whole size, check your foot doesn't slide around too much in the shoe as this can also cause blisters. A good rule of thumb is to actually use your thumb to find the correct fit – you should have a thumb's width between your big toe and the front of the shoe.

Depending on how much you run, your trainers should last at least a year before they need to be replaced. Many shoe manufacturers advise replacing a pair after running 500 miles in them, but make the judgement yourself based on whether they have worn down or lost their comfort and bounce.

Every woman knows you can never have too many shoes and when it comes to trainers, there are plenty of options to tempt you if you feel one pair isn't enough! You can easily manage with just one set, but if you want to take your training a bit more seriously you could swap to a lightweight pair for speed sessions and races, as having lighter feet can make you feel like you can run faster. If you want to run off-road, trail shoes are best as they have extra grip, and some are waterproof to keep your feet dry as you splash through mud and long, wet grass.

Barefoot running, which involves running without anything on your feet at all, or wearing very minimal trainers, is favoured by some runners who say it allows for a more natural running style. They believe modern trainers have too much cushioning, which forces people to heel strike as they land instead of landing on the forefoot, and that this means they run less efficiently and are more likely to develop injuries. However, barefoot running is also not without some injury risk, particularly when transitioning from a cushioned to a barefoot shoe. Some find that the lack of a shock absorber when striking the ground, particularly when landing on concrete, can cause sore feet and lead to stress fractures. If you're considering barefoot running, seek advice from an expert first.

TRAINER TALK

The choice of trainers can be mind-boggling. It's advisable to go to a specialist running shop for advice on the right shoe for your running style when you are starting out, but you might find some of the terminology they use even more confusing! Here's a guide to help.

▶**Gait analysis:** This is when running shop staff assess how your foot lands when you run to work out which type of trainer is best for you. They might be able to do this by just watching you run a few steps. Alternatively, some shops have treadmills hooked up to computers that can work it all out after you have run for a couple of minutes on them. Staff will tell you if you're a neutral runner or one who overpronates or underpronates.

▶**Neutral trainers:** These shoes are designed for those whose foot lands evenly on the floor when running. If you haven't had gait analysis or advice on your running style, it's best to go for this type of shoe when you are starting out.

▶**Underpronators:** The feet of underpronators, aka supinators, roll outward when striking the ground. Such runners often have a higher foot arch and should opt for cushioned trainers in the neutral category, avoiding 'stability' trainers that are designed for overpronators (see below).

▶**Stability trainers:** These are recommended for runners who 'overpronate', which means their foot rolls excessively inwards as they land. Trainers for overpronators have extra cushioning and 'motion control' so that, when this happens, the foot is supported and running is more comfortable. If you find running in neutral shoes makes your feet and lower legs sore, it's worth checking if shoes with extra stability would be more suitable.

▶**Lightweight shoes:** An obvious one, these are less bulky trainers made with light materials so your feet don't feel as heavy when running. They're often referred to as racing shoes or 'flats'. Many prefer to save running in such lightweight trainers for speed work and racing, as they find that they don't have enough support and cushioning to wear them on every run.

▶**Barefoot shoes:** Some runners prefer to run without any trainers on at all, but this isn't practical for all of us. Flat and light-soled barefoot trainers mean you still have something on your feet to offer a little protection from landing on stones, etc. but they have little or no cushioning.

▶ **Trail shoes:** These have extra grip and ankle support to aid running over slippery and uneven off-road terrain. These are a recommended buy if you intend to do fell or cross country running.

▶ **Spikes:** These are light trainers with holes in the sole to insert small spikes into for extra grip. Track runners wear short spikes, while cross country runners have longer ones for particularly muddy courses. If you're only planning on road running/racing you shouldn't need to buy any and, on many off-road courses, you can also get by with trail shoes.

▶ **Socks:** Specialist running socks are another essential item for optimum foot health. Not only are they designed to prevent blisters caused by rubbing, but they're made from air-wicking material, which means your feet don't get too damp when you sweat which can also help prevent blisters as well as athlete's foot.

▶ **Sports bra:** Do not run without one of these, ladies! Not only will they protect your breasts from sagging, they will also reduce bounce making you feel much more comfortable as you run. If you don't run with a supportive bra, you can get shoulder and back pain as well as sore breasts. There are a number of brands on the market; RMR members often recommend those made by Shock Absorber, Freya Active and Panache. They all cater for large cup sizes, so don't let having an ample cleavage be a barrier to your running. Some sports bras are underwired and support the breasts by cupping each one, while others are designed to 'compress' your chest to prevent bounce. Try a few on and see what works best for you. Some stores will also offer sports bra fittings so you can ensure you're running in the right size. It shouldn't be so tight that it causes painful chafing or digs in into skin, but needs to be secure enough to prevent chest bounce.

▶**Breathable, comfortable running clothing:** With a few running wardrobe staples you can run all year round. As well as a sports bra, all you need for your top half is a vest, a couple of T-shirts and a long-sleeved top or two and you can layer up according to the temperature outside. Go for products made from technical, breathable fabrics, as these are lightweight and wick sweat away from the body so your skin doesn't get cold and clammy. Unless it is a compression top which is designed to be skin-tight to increase blood flow to the muscles, pick a size that's a loose fit. This will enable you to move without feeling restricted and make it less likely to chafe under the arms. On your bottom half, go for garments made from stretchy material like Lycra to give you freedom of movement. If you have to be frugal, all you really need are shorts for the summer and leggings for the winter. Three-quarter length leggings (capris) that stop just below the knee are an additional wise buy for the days when the weather means you need something in between. They are also a good choice if you want to stay cooler and don't have the confidence to wear shorts. The RMR shop has another solution for this too – our super 'skort'. This is a running skirt with built-in shorts. It's really popular with our members who want to feel more feminine or keep a bit more covered up when running in the summer.

▶ **High-vis clothing:** As covered in the safety section (page 26), it is imperative to be visible to drivers when running after dark, so if you aren't able to run during daylight hours, you need high-vis, reflective clothing. You don't need to go mad and buy whole outfits of reflective clothing – you could just buy a high-vis running bib that you can pull on over your usual kit. White T-shirts and long-sleeved tops will also help you stand out, so go for these over dark shades if more of your running will be at night or early in the morning.

PRODUCTS YOU COULD RUN WITHOUT (BUT SHOULD GET ANYWAY!)

▶ **Compression socks:** Tightly-fitted compression socks worn over the calves are a huge talking point on the RMR Facebook group. It is believed that compression socks can help your running and recovery, and some say that, when worn during a run, they make their legs feel less heavy and tired. There's no conclusive evidence to prove that they can actually boost your performance, but, whether the effect is physical or psychological, if the socks make your legs feel better then you're more likely to run well. Where the evidence is more convincing is how compression socks can help your muscles recover after activity. They have been proven to help prevent DOMS (delayed onset muscle soreness – the aches and pains that can be felt after exercise) and reduce inflammation. As a result, some of our members only wear them post run.

Whenever you wear them, compression socks (and footless sleeves which just cover the calves) should be worn against the skin as the snug fit increases blood flow to the muscles. Some RMR members have asked if they can be worn under full-length leggings but we don't recommend this as the socks could then feel too tight. They are best worn with shorts or capris to be most comfortable. Wearing compression socks is definitely a matter of personal choice, so they are not a must-have item. Aside from any potential physical benefits, some of our members just love to wear them because of the colourful, funky designs!

▶ **Gadgets:** There are so many gadgets on the market, from pedometers to heart-rate monitors and GPS watches, it can be confusing knowing which, if any, are suitable for your needs.

▶ **Pedometers:** Knowing how many steps you've taken during a run isn't a necessity, but if it is something you're keen to know to stay motivated, opt for a pedometer. Choose one that also has a stopwatch and measures the distance you've covered so that you won't need to have a separate gadget if you want to start measuring your running time/distance (although the latter won't be quite as accurate as when using a GPS watch).

▶ **Heart rate monitors:** This gadget measures your number of heartbeats per minute either via a band worn around your chest or via a sensor on a wristwatch. Knowing your heart rate can aid your training because once you have worked out your maximum, you can push yourself to it when doing hard sessions and races. Knowing your heart rate can also help you tell if you are under the weather (if so it will be higher than usual on an easy run) and help you control your effort if running when pregnant. So knowing your heart rate certainly has its benefits, but it's not essential so there's no need to splash out on one if you can't afford it.

▶ **GPS watch:** A GPS watch links to a satellite to tell you the pace you're running at and the distance you've covered, so it's a great training aid. It can help you judge your pace so you don't begin too fast, and it can be a source of motivation when you see how you are improving. The data can be downloaded to a computer or mobile so you can keep a virtual training diary and share your routes and achievements with others. GPS watches are well-worth investing in – Garmin and TomTom are among some of the popular brands in the RMR community – but they aren't the be-all and end-all if you're on a tight budget. To begin with, any device that you can use to time your run will be fine.

Some RMR members prefer to run or race without the pressure of knowing how far they have gone, or at what speed. They just want to run based on how they feel, not based on information they are getting from their watch. Running this way – without using a gadget – has become known as going 'naked'. So, if you are invited on a naked run, remember: it's just your watch you need to leave at home and not the rest of your clothes!

▶**Running belts and rucksacks:** Running belts are great for carrying your mobile and keys on training runs. You can also get ones capable of carrying water bottles and energy gels when covering long distances. However, you can manage without one, particularly on short runs where you don't need to take water and gels, as some kit comes with zip-up pockets which you can use to secure your valuables instead. Alternatively, you can thread your key through your trainer lace and double knot it to carry it that way. When racing, there are usually water stations on the course, and in the case of half and full marathons, energy drinks and gels are sometimes handed out so you don't need to carry your own.

Running rucksacks are useful if you want to run-commute. They are designed with wide straps to stop your shoulders getting sore and to reduce the bag bouncing on your back. If you do run with a belt or bag, beware of over-packing it and weighing yourself down!

▶**Winter accessories:** When temperatures plummet there's no excuse not to keep running thanks to the plethora of warming accessories. Running thermal tops, hats, gloves and snugs (a lightweight neck scarf) are light and breathable so they will keep out the chill without making you feel too hot once you get running. With the exception of days when it is mega-freezing, you could manage without these products, as you soon warm up once you get going. But having these items will make you much more likely to go for a run when it's cold outside so they're well worth having for the winter months.

▶**Summer accessories:** When the heat is on, wear a vest to keep you cooler, a baseball cap to shield your face from the sun and sunglasses to protect your eyes. Buy the latter from a sports shop: you might find a 'normal' pair of sunglasses uncomfortable to run in, as they could bounce on your nose. A sporty pair will wrap around your face for a snug fit and have a high level of UV protection. Sweatbands on the wrists or worn as a headband are also useful to mop your brow with. You could manage without these items if you avoid running in the heat of the day when it's hot, but never forget to lather on suncream before you go for a run in the sun if the UV rays are strong.

DEFINITELY DITCH

▶ **Un-waterproof waterproofs:** If you don't want to let the weather rain on your running parade then a waterproof jacket is essential. It will keep you dry and warm, and if you also don a baseball cap to shield the droplets from your eyes, you'll soon forget it's even raining as you run. But beware of cheap products that claim to be waterproof but are actually just a flimsy, plastic layer. These products will quickly absorb water and cling to your skin making you feel like a drowned rat. A good waterproof jacket will be made from durable material, such as Gore-tex, and you'll be able to see the droplets of water repelled on the surface. However, you still need a product that is breathable or else you'll find you get hot and sweaty underneath the jacket and be soaking wet regardless. So ditch any waterproof that's too flimsy and isn't breathable. This is one accessory that is well worth spending a little extra on to ensure it is fit for purpose so you can happily run in the rain.

▶ **Uncomfortable trainers:** As stated in the earlier section on trainers (page 39), the right fit for you will depend on a number of factors including your running style, the terrain you will mostly run on and whether you prefer to have more or less cushioning. Much like finding your ideal partner, you may have to go through a process of trial and error before you find your perfect match! When you do find them you'll be so proud you'll want to show them off. RMR members share pictures of their favourite new trainers on the page so much it has cheekily been dubbed 'shoe porn'. Whenever you buy new trainers, it will take a little while to break them in so they feel comfortable (which is why it is not recommended to do a race in new shoes). But if, after a few wears, you still find they are rubbing painful blisters, making your feet feel sore or are giving you any niggling pain in your ankles or legs, it might be best to cut your losses and try a different pair rather than soldiering on (no matter how much you love how they look!). If they are too worn to get an exchange from the shop where you purchased them you could sell them second-hand, or keep them to wear for walking or going to the gym.

▶**Frequent consumption of sugary energy drinks:** Runners are often bombarded with information on nutritional products that will boost their energy and help them run faster. Such products can help if you are running a long distance but that doesn't mean you should be guzzling energy drinks during and after every training run. Energy drinks are often packed with sugar – and we all know that having too much of the sweet stuff is bad for our health as it can cause tooth decay and lead to weight gain and type 2 diabetes. So, unless you are running a long distance, save your money and your health by just sticking to drinking tap water as it will hydrate you without giving you a needless sugar rush. It's the same for recovery after a run. Protein can aid muscle repair but instead of spending on costly protein shakes and bars, just have some food and drink that's naturally high in protein, such as a glass of milk, nuts, eggs or cheese.

CHAPTER TWO:
RUN, WALK, RUN

JUST JEFF IT

RMR members often talk about 'Jeffing' to get fit or how they 'Jeffed' a marathon. New recruits often end up asking what they are talking about! Jeffing is an abbreviation of the name Jeff Galloway and has been coined as a verb by members who advocate the American's 'Run Walk Method'. Former Olympic athlete Jeff developed his run-walk-run schedules in 1973 when he turned his attention to coaching. As he tried to help beginners get fit, he found strategic walking breaks enabled them to fight fatigue and lessen their chance of getting injured. Often, novice runners will go out hard and then tire and give up after a few minutes. 'Jeffing' means they can pace themselves and set manageable targets. It's a lot easier to keep running for five minutes then walk for two minutes and repeat four times (to run a total of 20 minutes), than it is to run for 20 minutes continuously when you have never run for that long before.

Jeff, who has written numerous articles and books on running, has discovered that his method doesn't just help beginners. Many of his athletes achieve personal best times by having planned walking breaks during races compared to when they try to run all the way from start to finish. This has been backed up by numerous scientific studies, including one that found that intervals of walking allowed non-elite race participants to achieve similar finishing times to their peers who ran the whole way, with the added bonus of suffering from less muscle discomfort. Many competitors still prefer to run the entire distance of a race, but this study proves there's no shame in taking walking breaks, and it could be beneficial to your finishing time and experience.

Thousands of RMR members have found they have been able to take up and keep running thanks to following Jeff's advice, which is why he has become such a legend in the community. So, if you want to start running or get a PB, get Jeffing!

RUNNING FORM AND FLYING FEET!

If you're struggling to keep running for more than a minute when you're starting out, it might be that you are trying too hard and going too fast. It shouldn't be a sprint but a jog. You should still have enough breath to hold a conversation.

Focus on running at a pace you can sustain first, then you can consider going faster as you get fitter (you'll notice a natural progression with this anyway as your body adapts).

Think about your running form too to aid your movement. Your shoulders should be loose with your arms by your side, bent at the elbows. Try not to clench your fists or hunch your shoulders as this will make you tighten up. Don't drag your feet, try to get a little knee lift and aim to land each step under your hips rather than overstriding. RMR members love it when they get a running picture to prove they've perfected this, which shows them with 'flying feet'. This is when they are captured mid-stride with space between the ground and their about-to-land foot.

You might find that running doesn't come naturally at first, but you will start to find your form as you get fitter. Doing regular strengthening and core stability exercises like 'the plank' will help improve your posture and, in turn, your running action too (see page 82 for examples of exercises).

Once you're used to running you could also start doing some 'strides' occasionally to help improve your running form. Strides involve accelerating over a very short distance, such as 50–100 metres, and are usually done as part of a warm-up or towards the end of an easy run. They help you to focus on your form as you should be moving dynamically and driving the arms and legs like a sprinter. You can then do this at the very end of a race with a sprint finish where you work all the way to the line! Strides are often done along with other running 'drills' as part of a warm-up and to improve running form (see more on this in the glossary).

THE COUCH TO 5K PLAN

Jeff Galloway's method of walk-running has now become a universally accepted way to get fit, with many starting out by following a Couch To 5k plan (abbreviated to C25K). There are a number of these plans available and they can be downloaded as apps. Some aim to have you running 5k (3.1 miles) after six weeks, while others build up to the distance after eight or nine weeks. All involve running intervals with walking in between, gradually increasing the length of running time until you can manage 5k continuously.

If you think you will struggle to stay motivated to complete the course then search online, in local newspapers or by using the England Athletics directory at www.runtogether.co.uk/groups/ to find a running group in your area. Many will follow C25K plans and will arrange to meet up every week to do the runs. You could also form your own group by seeing if friends and family want to follow the schedule with you. Another way to stay motivated is to aim to do the 5k at the end of the plan as part of a fun run like parkrun, The Colour Run or Race For Life (see more on these events in the 5k section in chapter five). There's no pressure to run a certain time at these events and you'll be surrounded by other runners to pull you along. The atmosphere and adrenaline rush you'll get beforehand will also make doing your first 5k feel like more of an event rather than just another run.

The C25K plans found on the NHS, Bupa and Zenlabs websites are popular with the majority of RMR members. Public Health England have kindly allowed us to reproduce a version of their schedule here, a similar schedule can also be found online at www.nhs.co.uk or downloaded as an app called the 'One You Couch To 5k' on any smartphone. The latter provides step-by-step instructions telling you when to run and when to take a break, and you can even select a celebrity to narrate your journey. This plan involves running three times a week for nine weeks. We've outlined it here with runs on Mondays, Wednesdays and Saturdays, but the plan is flexible so you can fit the training in on the days it's most convenient for you. The main thing is to do three runs throughout the week with a rest day between each. We've added the total time each run-walk session takes to help you factor it into your day, followed by comments from RMR members on how they found it to give you help and encouragement along the way.

	Mon	Tue	Wed	Thur	Fri	Sat	Sun
Week 1	Walk 5 min. Run 1 min, walk 90 sec x 7. Run 1 min. Walk 5 min. Total: 28 min, 30 sec	Rest	Repeat week 1 Monday session	Rest	Rest	Repeat week 1 Monday session	Rest
Week 2	Walk 5 min. Run 90 sec, walk 2 min x 5. Run 90 sec. Walk 5 min. Total: 29 min	Rest	Repeat week 2 Monday session	Rest	Rest	Repeat week 2 Monday session	Rest
Week 3	Walk 5 min, run 90 sec, walk 90 sec, run 3 min, walk 3 min, run 90 sec, walk 90 sec, run 3 min, walk 3 min. Total: 23 min	Rest	Repeat week 3 Monday session	Rest	Rest	Repeat week 3 Monday session	Rest
Week 4	Walk 5 min, run 3 min, walk 90 sec, run 5 min, walk 2.5 min, run 3 min, walk 90 sec, run 5 min, walk 5 min. Total: 31 min, 30 sec	Rest	Repeat week 4 Monday session	Rest	Rest	Repeat week 4 Monday session	Rest

Week	Mon	Tue	Wed	Thur	Fri	Sat	Sun
Week 5	Walk 5 min. Run 5 min, walk 3 min x 2. Run 5 min. Walk 5 min. Total: 31 min	Rest	Walk 5 min, run 8 min x 2. Walk 5 min. Total: 31 min	Rest	Rest	Walk 5 min, run 20 min, walk 5 min. Total: 30 min	Rest
Week 6	Walk 5 min, run 5 min, walk 3 min, run 8 min, walk 3 min, run 5 min, walk 5 min. Total: 34 min	Rest	Walk 5 min, run 10 min, walk 3 min, run 10 min, walk 5 min. Total: 33 min	Rest	Rest	Walk 5 min, run 25 min, walk 5 min. Total: 35 min	Rest
Week 7	Repeat week 6 Saturday session	Rest	Repeat week 6 Saturday session	Rest	Rest	Repeat week 6 Saturday session	Rest
Week 8	Walk 5 min, run 28 min, walk 5 min. Total: 38 min	Rest	Repeat week 8 Monday session	Rest	Rest	Repeat week 8 Monday session	Rest
Week 9	Walk 5 min, run 30 min, walk 5min. Total: 40 min	Rest	Repeat week 9 Monday session	Rest	Rest	Do 5k run/ race	Rest

BEFORE YOU GO: TIPS FROM RMR MEMBERS ON STARTING C25K

'Use a flat route! Also, follow the same circuit each time. That way you know you've done it before, so you know mentally you can do it again.'

Sabah Moran

'I would definitely recommend doing it with someone else, even if it's just you and a friend rather than an organised group.'

Helen Spencer

'Run more slowly than you think. It isn't about going as fast as you can, it is about running for the set time. If it feels like you are going too fast and can't cope, then slow down.'

Paula Sheridan

'If you can't talk, you're going too fast!'

Nicola Bedford

'I joined a running group specifically for C25K, as when I tried on my own I couldn't find the motivation. Some runs are tough but don't give up!'

Jess Nelmes-Cook

'I refused to look at what came next. For someone who can talk themselves out of anything, this tactic works well.'

Joanna Brocklehurst Smith

'I found a route I enjoyed and ran two of the three runs each week on it. Then I made the third run a chance to explore for a change of scenery.'

Emily Linka Swiatek

'Don't compare yourself to others. Do your best.'

Mustang Sally

'Reward yourself for completing each week so you have minor targets to help you along the journey.'

Lorraine McDonald

'Believe in yourself because you CAN do it!'

Alyson Young

KEEP GOING! HOW RMR MEMBERS
MANAGED TO STICK TO THE PLAN

'I followed the plan with friends. At the end of week two we screamed, "OMG we just ran a mile without stopping!" It was a pivotal moment in our C25k journey.'

Elaine Diffenthal

'Week five, run three, don't doubt yourself – YOU CAN DO IT, and when you do you'll feel like you can do anything.'

Emma Forth

'Don't give up. For me, it took three attempts to finish the course, and weeks three to four were my killers. But after that it's just one foot in front of the other.'

Shell Teague

'If, at week three, you feel you're not ready to move to the next week, repeat the same week as many times as you feel you need to. For me it was about not giving up. By week five I'd found my stride.'

Louisa Middleweek

'Week eight, day one was my toughest run. Twenty-eight minutes without stopping. I was ready to give it all up but I stuck with it and completed the course. Now I feel so proud!'

Caroline Pocock

'At the start, I remember thinking I couldn't run for a minute and I really struggled. Then, around week five, my fitness level went up and things started to click. Now I'm not phased about running for fifteen minutes or even twenty-five minutes!'

Dominique Thorpe

WHAT A FEELING! RMR MEMBERS ON FINISHING THE SCHEDULE

'When I started the C25K, I never thought I'd run more than 5k, and now I want to run a half marathon! C25K showed me that I could do a lot more than I thought.'

Sarah Beeley

'When you run 5k for the first time, don't worry if it takes you longer than thirty minutes. It's about the distance and building strength and stamina.'

Sarah Angela Bentley

'When I joined my local C25K group I was massively overweight and had never run before. I lost a pound a week on the course and haven't looked back! I am now a stone lighter and the leader of my very own C25K group.'
Rebecca Pass

'I never doubted the plan. I stuck to it even on holiday. Running 5k was incredible. Just amazing. I still laugh when I realise I run. C25K works.'
Kirsty Jayne

'When I started C25K, I didn't really think I'd finish it. But it was easy to follow and I could really see my progress, so I just kept going. It's definitely one of the best things I've ever done.'
Lucy Parrett

RMR STORIES

'Sticking with the C25K plan paid off!': RMR's Hannah Hiscock, 35, from Swindon, Wiltshire, thought she would never be a bona fide runner after failing to complete the C25K plan the first time she attempted it. She tried again and now she's not just gone from Couch to 5k... but to ultra-marathon!

The first time I attempted the C25K plan it didn't go well. I quit three weeks in because I lost motivation and found it so tough.

Then a year later I heard there was going to be a Colour Run 5K held just ten minutes away from my house. The carnival-like event, where you are splattered with colourful dye along the route, looked like so much fun. I knew I had to try the C25K plan again so I would be fit enough to take part. I persuaded a neighbour, Julie, to do it with me and having her company and support helped immensely – we were in it together.

Doing the C25K plan this time around I felt amazing from the very first session. I felt like I was making a difference to my fitness and it was the first step towards achieving my goal of completing The Colour Run. Targeting the race made a huge difference to my motivation. There was never any doubt in my mind this time that I wouldn't see the plan through until the end, as I was so determined to take part in the event.

There were plenty of times I still found it hard though and Julie and I weren't confident in our abilities. We often referred to ourselves as 'two unfit girls' and to other runners we saw as 'proper runners'. We went out at night in the dark dressed in jogging bottoms and hoodies praying that no one we knew would spot us! We were absolutely mortified when a friend drove past and beeped!

After walk-running for a few weeks as outlined by the programme, we managed to start getting faster and were able to keep running for longer.

Then the day of The Colour Run arrived and I was so excited to take part. The run isn't timed so there was no pressure to go at a certain pace or worry about the finishing time. It was all about the achievement of getting round and enjoying it. The race met all my expectations and I had a fantastic day. I couldn't believe it when I crossed the finish line. I was tired, my legs were sore but I felt amazing – I had completed a 5k run! I was so glad I had stuck with the C25K training plan and it had paid off.

After that there was no looking back and I moved on to the next challenge! I've now done 10ks, trail runs, a half marathon, a full marathon and even an ultra.

I would say to anyone thinking of doing the C25K plan that I wasn't born an athlete, and if I can become a runner, you can too. It didn't come easily to me, but I am strong-willed, so the day I signed up to The Colour Run was the day I knew I wouldn't quit. Find something that will motivate you to stick with it.

I'd also recommend joining the RMR group for support. I stumbled across it when I was searching for running groups on Facebook, as once I was committed to the C25K plan, I had a real thirst for knowledge and wanted to learn as much as I could about running. RMR immediately struck me as the most caring and supportive community, and I was hooked. RMR is in my blood now – I can't get enough of giving back to the community that helped me so much, so I volunteered to become one of the page admins and a community manager for one of the regional groups.

I've also helped as a volunteer with a free C25K group run by my local Be Active Group. I regularly tell runners that I started exactly where they are, and I've discovered I am capable of so much more than I once thought.

OTHER WAYS TO GET STARTED

While many RMR members have found the C25K plan has helped them immensely, there are lots of other options if you feel it's not for you. For instance, if you are doing a road run, instead of running for a set length of time, you could try running the distance between lamp posts, then walking between the next two, and so on. Wendy Marsh is one of the RMR members who said her preference was to start alone without a training plan, group or technology. She said: 'I just went out one evening and tried. I hadn't heard of any apps, I just had a pair of trainers and some determination. I walked, I ran, I walked some more. I enjoyed it but I wondered how on earth people ran more than a few hundred metres! I went again and again and when I was brave enough to tell my sister what I was doing, she told me about parkrun.

So that became my goal. I chose a date we could both go and aimed for that. I have never looked back, and I did my first half marathon within the year. And all because I decided to put on my trainers and try. Looking back now, I liked it my way – no one telling me when to walk and when to run, just going with how I felt.'

Meanwhile, Rachael Oldfield found plotting a route around a local field helped her. She said: 'It started as a challenge to run-walk around the field once, then twice, then three times. I then built up to running all the way around three times. It was then I decided to measure the distance on a running app and found the loop was 1k. I started to run five laps within weeks and a love was born! I've gone on to run a half marathon and I've also started marathon training.'

Whether you decide to follow the C25K plan or make up your own run-walk routine, build up the running sections gradually. If you are struggling, remember that nobody gets fit overnight.

Hang in there and you will start to see an improvement and feel fitter after regularly running three times a week. And, if you can't find anyone to run with, remember you still don't have to do it alone. Share your journey in the RMR group and you will get buckets of support and encouragement.

C25K ACCOMPLISHED – WHAT NEXT?
HOW TO KEEP IMPROVING

Running can be very addictive and once you've experienced the euphoria of finishing your first 5k, you are bound to be keen to do more. So, what's next? After reaching the 5k milestone, you might decide you want to try to go faster or further (or both!). If you enjoyed sticking to a set schedule like the C25K provided, then you can find 10k, half and marathon plans at the back of the book which are designed to follow on from it. Here are some more tips on how to keep improving.

▶**parkrun regularly:** If there's one near you, you might have already aimed for a parkrun at the end of your C25K plan, but if you haven't joined in one yet then now is the time! The events are held every Saturday at 9 a.m. in parks across the UK and around the world. As they are held every week, it will be easy for you to keep your training momentum going after finishing the C25K if you attend regularly. As well as it counting as one of your weekly runs, you'll also be able to meet other local runners there. Find out more about parkrun in the 5k event section on page 145.

▶**Enter a race:** Once you've got used to running, why not challenge yourself to do a race? Having a goal to work towards can really motivate you to train. It doesn't have to be a long-distance event like a marathon – there are plenty of other options, from 5ks to half marathons.

Racing will give you the opportunity to run with hundreds, if not thousands, of others and feel part of the friendly running community. Finishing a race will give you a huge sense of achievement, and you'll feel like an Olympian when you're cheered all the way round the course by spectators.

Even better, the majority of races give out medals at the finish so you'll have some bling to reward your effort!

Check out the 'Race Mummy Race' chapter (page 142) later in the book for more on racing, including recommended events and race day tips.

▶ **Vary your running routes:** Once you are feeling more confident about running, start exploring some new routes near where you live. If you have been sticking to the same road-run round the block this could soon become boring and uninspiring. Try going off-road so you can run surrounded by beautiful countryside and take in some hills to give you extra leg strength.

▶ **Increase your distance:** If you want to be able to run beyond 5k then gradually start increasing the length of one of your weekly runs by five minutes each week. In order to avoid injury, it's always best to gradually increase your mileage rather than jumping straight from running 30 minutes to an hour. The sky is the limit when it comes to how far you want to run, but do remember that the longer you carry on the more stress you are putting on your body, and you will need more time to recover afterwards. Most runners will only do one long run a week, capping the distance according to their goals.

▶ **Run more than three times a week:** If you have time, increase your number of runs to four per week. As you get fitter and stronger, up your training to run five or six times a week if you want to see even further improvements to your fitness. You don't have to go far or work hard each time to see results. It's not advisable to run every day of the week though, as a rest day (or days) give your body a chance to recuperate.

However, on occasion, some RMR members enjoy 'streaking' to stay motivated. Don't worry, you can keep your clothes on to do it! It involves achieving a 'running streak' by going every day for a certain length of time, such as a fortnight. While 'streaking' can keep you motivated, we'd only recommend doing it occasionally and not for long periods as it is very important to have days off to avoid injury and burnout. Also, remember to listen to your body: don't go out running if you feel poorly just for the sake of keeping a 'streak' going.

▶ **Join a running club:** Many running or athletics clubs that don't cater for absolute beginners will be open to you once you can run 5k. Joining a club will help you maintain a routine and increase your fitness levels, and you might even find you're faster than you thought as you start competing on friendly terms with other members of the group. They might also enter local races, and you could find it's more fun to participate as part of a club than on your own. Clubs are also full of experienced runners and coaches who can support you and give you advice as you continue your running journey.

▶ **Speed up:** Chasing a personal best time is what motivates many to keep running. As the name suggests, it's not about being the fastest but about being the best you can be – it's a personal goal.

As you get fitter, you'll soon find you start to get progressively faster but then you might plateau. If, at that point, you want to improve your pace then you'll need to start doing some speed work once or twice a week. Not only will this kind of training make you quicker, it will also burn more calories and add variety to your training. If you do speed work, make sure you take it easy the following day to give your body a chance to recover, as you might suffer from DOMS (delayed onset muscle soreness – see the glossary, page 248) from pushing yourself harder than usual.

Below are a number of options to keep you fit and interested when it comes to improving your pace. Make sure you precede any of these runs with a warm-up jog, and follow them with a cool-down jog of five to ten minutes to avoid injury.

> ▶ **Interval training:** This is very much like doing the C25K again with periods of running being interspersed with walking or jogging to recover, e.g. 3x five-minute runs with 90 seconds for recovery between each repetition, 7x two-minute runs with one minute for recovery. However, this time the running parts need to be as fast as you can go – if you have the breath to talk, then you aren't pushing yourself enough! It will be a learning curve to work out how to pace yourself throughout the whole session, and it will hurt! But this is a case of no pain, no gain. Such interval sessions will raise your heart rate, make you breathe harder and help you burn more calories in a similar way to a HIIT (high intensity interval training) gym class. During the

sections where you are running hard you need to be able to run without stopping, so it's best to find an area where you can do this safely without having to cross roads etc. Hence, many clubs will organise these kinds of sessions on a track. You could also run on grass around a park or lake, or go along a pedestrianised path. If you haven't done interval training before, start by doing fewer reps and then build them up gradually as you get fitter.

▶ **Hill reps:** These will improve your strength and stamina as well as your speed. Do repetitions by running up a hill hard and then jogging back down again.

▶ **Fartlek:** As comical as it sounds, this has nothing to do with breaking wind! It's a Swedish word meaning 'speed play' and involves running at different paces throughout a run in an unstructured way. As you go along, you can decide when you want to run faster and for how long. So you might decide to have a burst of speed for a certain number of minutes with a jog in between, e.g. running hard for one minute, running easy for one minute, repeated five times. Or you can measure your bursts of speed by distance instead, e.g. by running hard to a certain point you can see up ahead, such as a bench. Some RMR members set up timed intervals on their watches or run hard between two lamp posts, then easy between the next two lamp posts, and so on. The idea is you end up injecting some faster paced periods into your run without it feeling as serious as an interval session.

▶ **Paarlauf:** This is a way to do some speed work with a friend – the word means 'pairs' in German. You might find you're more motivated to push yourself if you're not alone. The sessions involve one of you running hard while the other jogs and then you switch places, doing this for a set length of time e.g. 20 minutes. Traditionally it is done on a track where one person runs hard round the bend and the other jogs across the middle and then you swap places. You could do a similar loop around a playing field, or one of you could run out and back to the same point for a minute while the other jogs on the spot. This is a good option if you have small children in buggies with you, as one of you will always stay with them while jogging.

▶ **Tempo runs:** Also known as threshold running, this involves going at a faster pace than you would go at on an easy run – but not as flat out as when you are doing intervals – for a predetermined time/distance. It should be around 70–80 per cent of your maximum capacity, so it shouldn't feel completely comfortable and you shouldn't be able to hold a conversation, but you should feel like it's a pace you could keep going at beyond a mile. The length of time you run at this pace for will be dependent on your goals. If you are targeting a 5k, then do a 10–20 minute tempo run, for a 10k 20–30 minutes etc. Learning what pace you can sustain over a longer distance will really help you when it comes to racing and pushing yourself to run a PB.

CHAPTER THREE:
HOW TO KEEP ON RUNNING (AND KNOW WHEN TO TAKE A BREAK)

WHEN IT FEELS LIKE IT ISN'T GETTING ANY EASIER

When you first take up running and your fitness is low you're bound to find it difficult. You might be huffing and puffing, giving your all but still barely able to make it to a minute of continuous running. Then, when you see other runners zooming past and making it look easy, you might feel defeated and believe the problem must be you – that you're not cut out to be a runner. Well, firstly, remember that everyone has to start somewhere. That other runner bouncing by was once a beginner like you, and they got to where they are through dedication and patience. So don't give up. No one sees a huge leap in their fitness after one or two attempts, or even after one or two weeks of trying. If you keep it going you will soon start to reap the rewards. Many RMR members who followed the Couch To 5k plan said they noticed a difference in how they felt around week five of the nine-week plan. However, based on a variety of factors including your genes, build and age, everyone progresses differently, so don't compare yourself negatively to others, particularly if you are in a beginners' group and see some make breakthroughs in their fitness before you do.

Also, keep in mind that, no matter how fit someone is, they can still have days when they feel tired and sluggish. Running makes us feel fabulous the majority of the time, but everyone will have the occasional 'bad' run, so don't let an unsatisfying session make you feel like you can't do it or that you won't ever improve.

▶ **Know when to take a break:** Whether you're just starting to run or you're trying to get back into it after time off with injury or after childbirth, don't overdo it in a bid to get to where you want your fitness to be more quickly. Take the rest days advised in your schedule, or make sure you plot regular days off yourself if you aren't following a set plan. It might be tempting to think you'll get fitter faster if you go hell for leather and run as much as possible, but this is more likely to lead to you getting ill or injured. Rest days give your body a chance to repair, recover and adapt to the training you have done, which, in turn, will help you improve.

PREVENTING INJURY AND ILLNESS

Once you have discovered a love of running it's frustrating if you develop an injury that can prevent you doing it. Depending on the severity of the problem, you might need to take days, weeks or even months off to allow your body to recover. Prevention is better than a cure, so here are our tips to avoid getting sidelined:

▶ **Stretch and roll:** When you run regularly, your muscles can become tight and stiff. This can create all sorts of niggles, from aching knees to a very literal pain in the bum. When you're starting out, you might think such soreness is an injury that will prevent you running, but if it's just a tight muscle, you should find the pain eases off as you run and the muscle warms up. One way to alleviate this kind of muscle tightness is to stretch immediately after you have been running. Most of us don't have the time to do this after every run, but if you can, try to fit in five to ten minutes of stretching a couple of times a week. Going to a regular Pilates or yoga class will also help and you'll be led through the moves by an expert.

Another option to help remove tight spots from your muscles is to use a foam roller. These are cylindrical pieces of equipment that you can roll along your body to give yourself a massage. You can achieve a similar effect by rolling on a tennis ball. For example, one of the most common niggles in new runners is 'runner's knee'. This is when the IT band – connective tissue that runs up the outside of the thigh between the knee and hip – becomes tight. You can ease the pain by stretching and also by lying on a foam roller or tennis ball. Lie on the affected side and place the roller under the outside of your knee with your weight on it. Then push your body so the roller moves up the outside of your thigh to your hip joint. It will hurt at the time but should then feel much better afterwards as the tension will be released.

If your legs are particularly tight and sore and stretching and foam-rolling isn't making a great difference, visit a professional sports masseur. You can expect the treatment to be quite painful as opposed to relaxing as they will apply pressure to ease out your knots. You might still feel a little achy the following day, but after that you should feel much looser. An hour's massage can cost anything from £20–50 but you can find cheaper options if you shop around. Many money-saving websites have offers for sports massages. Alternatively, if there is a college near you where they teach it, they often need willing volunteers for students to practise on. You could also ask friends or family to buy vouchers for you to have a sports massage if they want to buy you a birthday or Christmas present. While it's not something you need to splash out on every month (unless you're doing very high mileage) it is money well spent as a treat once in a while, as it could help you avoid injury further down the line and make you feel like you have brand new legs!

EXAMPLE STRETCHES

Here are a few stretches you can do to ease muscle tension after running. Aim to hold each for 20–30 seconds.

▶**Quads:** Stand on one leg then bend the other leg up behind you so you're holding your foot in your hand. Your heel should be positioned close to your bottom. Hold, then repeat with the other leg. You should feel this stretching the quad muscle on the front of your thigh.

▶**Calves:** Stand facing one stride away from a wall and reach forward so your arms are outstretched, palms touching the wall. Place one foot forward and then bend that knee forward towards the wall, keeping both feet on the floor. You should feel the stretch in the calf muscle (lower back of the leg) of the straight leg. Hold and then repeat with the other foot forward.

▶**Hamstrings:** Find something to prop your leg on, like a low bench or garden wall. Stand up straight with one leg raised on the bench/wall. Lean forward slightly keeping the legs straight. You should feel this stretching the hamstrings (running along the back of the thigh) of the raised leg. Hold and repeat on the other leg.

▶ **Glutes:** Sit on the floor with your arms behind you to balance and then bend your left leg in front of you as if you are going to sit cross-legged. Then lift your right leg and bring it across the bent left leg to place the sole of the foot on the outside of the left thigh. Then use your left arm to hug the right knee to your chest while slightly twisting your body to look over your right shoulder, keeping your right arm behind you for balance. Hold and repeat with the other leg. You should feel this stretch in each buttock.

▶ **Warm up and cool down:** Every run on the C25K plan we published in chapter two (page 58) begins with a warm-up and cool-down walk, and this is a good habit to get into. Once you're fitter you don't have to walk to begin with but just run at a slightly slower pace to gradually raise your heart rate and get your body ready to exercise. Never do any sort of speed work or a hard race without warming up for at least ten minutes first, as otherwise you will be much more likely to pull a muscle. The cool-down is also important to reduce the severity of delayed onset muscle soreness (DOMS).

▶ **Build up mileage gradually:** Many runners sustain an injury because they do too much too soon. If you want to run further it's always best to up your training gradually, particularly if you are aiming for a long-distance race like a marathon. If it's your speed you are looking to improve, don't do hard interval sessions back-to-back as you need to give yourself time to recover from the effort. If you've had to take time off running due to illness or injury, make sure you return to training gradually as well to avoid ill-health or old injuries returning.

▶ **Take regular rest days:** Schedule at least one rest day a week into your running plans to give both your body and mind a break from training. It's also important to rest after doing a hard race, particularly a marathon, to allow yourself to recover – and have a chance to celebrate your achievement!

▶ **Cross train:** Other forms of exercise, like swimming and cycling, can improve your fitness and aid your running, while having less stress on your joints. Doing strength and conditioning exercises will also decrease your chance of getting injured as you are making your body stronger. If you can't get to the gym or afford membership, there are plenty of moves you can do for free inside your own home, such as squats and core stability exercises – see the box on page 82 for more details.

▶ **Think about your non-running footwear:** After spending ages finding perfect running shoes, don't ruin your efforts to stay injury-free by wearing uncomfortable shoes when you're not running. High heels and tight-fitting ballet pumps, which you might wear on a night out or at work, could cause problems that will stop you running. So apply the same rules when shoe-shopping as you do for trainer-shopping and go for ones which are not going to rub blisters, give you bunions or make your feet and legs ache.

EXERCISES TO STRENGTHEN YOUR LEGS, ARMS AND CORE

Personal trainer and mum of three Debbie Watts (www.molevalleyfitness.co.uk) recommends that runners do these exercises once or twice a week. They will enhance your strength and core stability, making you a stronger runner who is less likely to get injured.

▶**Squats:** This move will help strengthen your legs and core and tone your bottom.

Start by standing straight with your feet slightly wider than hip width apart, toes should point out slightly. Bend at the knees and lower your bottom as if you are going to sit on a chair – keep your chest up and your knees behind your toes – and stand up straight again. Look up at a fixed point in front of you rather than looking down as you do the move. Do three sets of five repetitions with 60–90 seconds between sets, building up to three sets of fifteen repetitions as you get stronger.

▶**Pistol squats from a chair:** Adding this move to your repertoire will improve balance and ankle strength.

Start by sitting on a chair with your back straight. One foot should be on the floor and the other should be raised slightly off the floor with the leg straight (beginners can start with this heel touching the floor and using the table for support). Rise up from the chair to standing, balance on one foot and then lower back down again. Repeat three sets of five repetitions with 60–90 seconds between sets, building up to three sets of fifteen repetitions as you get stronger.

▶**Reverse lunges:** This is another great move to improve leg strength, tone your bottom and strengthen your core. Watts recommends this version over the traditional forward-stepping lunge as it puts less strain on the knees.

Start in a standing position and imagine tramlines behind you. Keeping your back straight, step one foot back as if onto the tramline behind you and then lower to the floor bending both knees. Once the knee of your back leg is almost touching the floor, hold the position for a second and then rise back up to the standing position. Repeat with the other leg stepping back. If you have space, make them travelling lunges where you keep stepping back each time on alternate legs. Repeat three sets of five repetitions with 60–90 seconds between sets, building up to three sets of twenty repetitions as you get stronger.

▶ **Press ups:** These are known for improving upper-body strength but they also work the core so can aid your overall posture.

Beginners should start by resting on their knees on the floor at a 45-degree angle with their arms straight and palms flat on the floor (or can do it against a wall or kitchen worktop), positioned beneath the shoulders. Gently lower your body until your arms are bent at a 90-degree angle, then push back up again and repeat. Once you have mastered this, advance to starting with your toes on the floor and your legs and back straight as you do the move. Repeat three sets of five repetitions with 60–90 seconds between sets, building up to three sets of fifteen repetitions as you get stronger.

▶ **The bridge:** This position will strengthen your legs and tone your bottom, as well as improving your core stability.

Lie on your back with your knees bent and feet flat on the floor close to your bottom. Slowly lift your bottom off the floor, squeezing your glutes (bum muscles) and keeping your stomach held in, until your body is in a straight line. Hold the position then lower your bottom. Repeat ten times.

▶**Bridge clams:** This has the additional benefits from the bridge of improving hip rotation and activating the glutes. From the bridge position, bring the feet together, then open and close the legs, whilst keeping the bottom raised. Repeat ten times.

▶**Run off-road:** Not only is running on grass and trail paths more exhilarating, it could also reduce your risk of injury. This is because running on a surface softer than concrete is kinder to the joints, and the uneven surface of the grass can improve your ankle stability and leg strength.

▶**Know when to take a break:** If you experience any sharp pain that doesn't ease off then stop running. Listen to your body and learn when it's telling you it's just a bit tired and sore, and when carrying on running is actually a very bad idea. If you have persistent muscle pain after running, this is another sign that all is not well. If you suspect you have an injury then seek the help of a medical professional, such as a physiotherapist, who can advise you. They will be able to aid your recovery and identify the cause of the injury to prevent it returning again, e.g. they could give you some strengthening exercises for a specific muscle or muscle group that might be causing problems when you run because it is too weak. Being told you can't run when all you want to do is exercise can be annoying but if you don't rest when it's in your best interest, you could make a problem worse. Sometimes it is better to take a couple of days off to prevent having to take weeks or months off further down the line. If you are concerned about losing the fitness you have gained, you could see if you can do other forms of exercise instead such as walking, swimming or cycling.

It's the same if you are feeling poorly – don't push yourself to run if you are not up to it as you could make yourself worse. If you have a cold, a sore throat or a temperature, your body is fighting an infection or virus and needs all the energy it can get to recover.

Again, when it comes to illness, prevention is better than a cure. Try to get plenty of sleep and have regular days off running to stop you getting run-down. Eat lots of fruit and vegetables as the vitamins and minerals they contain will boost your health.

If you are unwell or are taking any medication, such as antibiotics, then do check with your doctor about how much exercise it's safe for you to do. Running should enhance your health, not endanger it.

COMMON RUNNERS' INJURIES
AND HOW TO DEAL WITH THEM

Here are a few of the most common problems runners experience, particularly when they first take up running. If you have any concerns about pains you're experiencing when running then seek advice from a medical professional.

▶ **Runner's knee:** Knee pain can be prevalent in those who first take up running, and research has found that women are twice as likely to get it than men (likely because we have wider hips). Running naysayers will, at this point, urge you to quit, telling you running is 'bad' for your knees and will lead to you getting arthritis. However, there is no evidence to prove the latter, and by avoiding running you will be missing out on all the other associated health benefits. Runner's knee shouldn't hold you back and can be easily treated. It is caused by the muscles around the knee cap becoming too tight and pulling it off-centre. To stop it developing in the first place, follow the injury prevention tips explained earlier in the book, including upping your mileage gradually (page 80), doing some runs off-road (page 85) and wearing the right trainers for your running gait (page 39). If you do develop an ache in your knee then regularly stretch your quads, hamstrings and IT band after running. Do some self-massage by using a foam roller or tennis ball (as explained in the 'stretch and roll' tip on page 77) to further release the tension, or see a sports masseur. Avoid running up hills until your knee feels better, and strengthen up your quads by doing moves such as squats. If none of this helps and you are still experiencing sharp pain, see a physiotherapist for further advice.

▶ **Plantar fasciitis:** This is a pain in the foot and heel caused when connective tissue in the area becomes inflamed – often due to running in inadequate shoes for your gait or doing too much running. For an initial treatment, ice the foot, regularly stretch your calf muscles and reassess the trainers you have been running in. You can self-massage the foot by rolling it over a tennis ball. This injury can be persistent so if icing, stretching, self-massaging and wearing the correct trainers hasn't helped, see a sports physio before it gets worse. They will be able to give you strengthening exercises, and might also recommend that you get orthotics (bespoke insoles to wear in your trainers when running).

▶ **Shin splints:** The muscles around your shin bones can often become sore if your calf muscles are too tight, you up your training too quickly, or if you frequently run on hard surfaces. If you have this problem, stretch regularly, ice the area after running if it becomes inflamed and try wearing compression socks during and after running. Run off-road as much as possible too, focusing on soft surfaces like grass until the discomfort eases.

If the pain is persistent, see a sports masseur or a physio for further treatment, as in some cases it could lead to a stress fracture.

▶ **Stress fractures:** This occurs when the repetitive force of running causes a slight fracture in the bone, but not a clean break. For runners, it is most likely to occur in the foot and shin bone after they have been doing high mileage, and particularly if a lot of it was on hard surfaces like concrete. The symptoms include a dull pain which can persist during and after exercise, and the area may become swollen and tender to touch. In most cases, rest will allow the body to mend and fuse the bone back together by itself, usually in about six to eight weeks. However, if it is severe a cast might be needed. Either way, to aid healing you will need to take a break from running and try to keep the weight off the injured area as much as possible. You could maintain fitness by doing other non-load-bearing exercise, such as swimming. To avoid this injury happening, it's important to keep your bones strong. Include plenty of calcium in your diet (found in milk, yoghurt, cheese, kale and almonds), do strengthening exercises like squats and consider lifting weights, as this has also been proven to improve bone density.

▶**Twisted ankle/pulled muscle:** If you hit an uneven surface when you land on your foot or have weak lower-leg muscles, you could go over on your ankle. If this happens, stop running, as carrying on could only make the pain and damage to your body worse. Once home, ice the area – a bag of frozen food will suffice if you don't have an ice pack, or you can wrap ice cubes in a tea towel. Icing will reduce the pain, swelling and inflammation. You could also take anti-inflammatories, such as ibuprofen, as long as they are suitable for you and you follow the manufacturers' instructions on dosage. Follow this procedure if you have experienced any other sprained muscle while running.

In the case of a twisted ankle, keep the ankle elevated to further reduce the swelling and pull on your compression socks or sleeves to further help with this. Rest until any swelling or pain has subsided. To strengthen the ankle once the swelling has gone, balance on the affected foot regularly. You could easily fit this in to your day, for example, by balancing while waiting for the kettle to boil. If you have pulled a muscle and the pain hasn't subsided by following the RICE procedure outlined here (Rest, Ice, Compression, Elevation), seek advice from an expert.

IF YOU GET A STITCH OR CRAMP

Getting a side stitch can be painful and debilitating when you're trying to run, and, unfortunately, they are more likely to afflict beginners than seasoned runners. They are felt when the diaphragm (a muscle under the lower ribs) cramps up because it is under increased pressure caused by rapid breathing. This is why novice runners often get them because their breathing can be more laboured. However, being super fit doesn't guarantee you'll never get one, as they can also strike after eating too close to exercising, or when doing speed work without an adequate warm-up. Some runners can also get a referral pain, where a stitch is felt in their shoulder.

Another common problem for runners is getting cramp in their legs and feet during or after running. It can be particularly agonising and make you feel like the whole muscle is seizing up. There isn't conclusive evidence on what causes cramp, but as it often strikes beginners, sprinters or those running long distances, fatigue is likely to be a factor due to the exertion of either running very fast, or for a long time. Some also believe it is caused by dehydration and salt depletion thanks to sweating. If these theories are correct then the best way to avoid cramp is to always do a good warm-up before exercise; prepare for long distances by building up to them gradually; and to stay hydrated before, during and after exercise.

Stomach cramps caused by period pain are another matter. See chapter four (page 125) for more information on this.

▶**Know when to take a break:** If you get a side stitch, slow down to a jog or walk and try to take in some big, deep breaths. If easing your pace doesn't make a difference, then stop completely and stretch your arms up as you inhale to get some more air into your lungs. The pain of a stitch is only temporary so it should pass once your breathing has regulated.

If you experience cramp, you might also find it difficult to carry on running. Some find walking and stretching can help, or that rubbing the muscle to increase blood flow to the area eases the pain. Have some water or an energy drink in case the cramp has been caused by dehydration.

WHEN MOTIVATION STARTS TO WANE

Even the most dedicated and enthusiastic runners can struggle with motivation at times. It might be due to work or family life getting in the way or when cold, dark winter months make getting out less appealing. Sometimes if you have achieved (or just missed out on) a target you've worked hard towards you can also feel flat and wonder what the point of carrying on is. So what can you do if you've lost your running mojo?

▶**Find what makes you happy:** RMR member Sara Spells has a fabulous tip to stay motivated. She says: 'Find what makes you happy, whether that's music, running with friends, running by the seaside or on trail, and do that. If you're happy then you will want to get out there week after week.'

▶**Keep track:** If you haven't already, start keeping a training diary. This could be by using good old pen and paper, digitally on your mobile or computer, or by keeping your own running blog. Knowing you have pages to fill in in your diary, or an audience to update via your blog, could make you much more motivated to go out. Looking back on what you have achieved should also keep you going.

▶**Set another goal:** If you are feeling demotivated because you have achieved a goal and now don't have anything to work towards then set yourself a new target. You could try aiming for a longer distance or running faster to beat your PB. Alternatively, if you're lacking in energy because a goal is proving too tricky, set something a little more manageable to work towards.

▶**Do something different:** If you've become bored of the same running routes then explore other options. Check out an Ordnance Survey map for your area and you might discover places and paths you didn't know were there. On occasion, you could also try taking a short drive to a new route, such as the coast, to give yourself a change of scenery. Try something different when it comes to racing too. If you've only done road runs, why not try a hilly and muddy cross country race or an obstacle course challenge?

▶ **Get a little help from your friends:** If you're struggling to stay motivated, let a friend know so they can help. It might just mean they send you a message to give you a kick up the bum to make you go when you said you would, or you could arrange to meet and run together. You'd be letting them down if you cancel, and it's much more fun with more than one.

▶ **Watch a race:** Marathon running legend Katherine Switzer once said: 'If you are losing faith in human nature, go out and watch a marathon.' It's true: watching others run and striving to achieve their goals can be very inspiring. This isn't just the case for marathon running either. If you are feeling demotivated, go along to another local race, to a parkrun or watch athletics coverage on TV. Seeing the dedication and determination of others is bound to make you want to chase your own dreams. If you want some company, then RMR regularly organise 'cheer squads' at major events like the London Marathon and Great North Run. By joining these squads, not only will you be offering much-needed support and encouragement to other runners, you'll also get to meet other RMR members and you'll find that their love of running is infectious. We guarantee you'll want to pull your trainers back on once you get home!

▶ **Know when to take a break:** Despite the best intentions, sometimes it isn't always possible to get out for a run or stick to a training schedule. Family commitments and busy or stressful situations, such as moving house, the school holidays, or caring for poorly children or elderly parents might mean you lack the energy, time or the will to go. You might be demotivated because you are simply exhausted and just need a break. If that's the case, don't feel guilty because you can always come back to it. As RMR member Paula Sheridan puts it: 'Running is like an old friend. You might go through periods where you don't see each other much, but it's always there. And always ready to welcome you back.'

WHEN YOU FEEL LIKE YOU'RE NOT IMPROVING

When you first take up running you can improve by leaps and bounds, finding your pace picking up and your fitness quickly improving. After a while, though, you might hit a plateau and find that, no matter how hard you try, you are not getting any faster.

If knocking time off your PB is your goal, you should try reassessing your training plan. Tempo/threshold runs, where you run a bit quicker, at 70–80 per cent of your maximum effort, will improve your speed endurance and help your body get used to running at a faster pace. Or, if you have only been doing easy-to-steady-paced runs, you could start introducing some regular speed sessions such as intervals and hill reps.

If you are keen to take your running more seriously, you could consider getting a coach. They are not just for elite runners: they could give you a personalised training plan and advise you on how to improve. Their support could also help you to keep going when it feels like you're stagnating. There might be a coach at your local running club who would be willing to help you, or there are plenty available online (but always double check their qualifications and experience in these cases). Then it is just a case of being patient, as if you have changed your training, you won't see improvements immediately.

Another way to improve your training is to be more focused on a certain race distance and tailor your training to it. For instance, if you want to do a faster 5k you need to do speed work once a week with short intervals of running fast with a brief recovery (for example running hard for two minutes with a minute jog recovery in between each, six times). In comparison, if it's the half marathon you want to excel at you need to do longer intervals in your speed sessions, such as running hard for five minutes with 90 seconds jog recovery, four times. You should also do tempo/threshold runs at your target race pace. For example, run easy for two miles, run the next two miles at your tempo pace, and then run two miles easy. You can find more examples of such sessions in the training plans at the back of the book.

▶**Know when to take a break**: You might be training your heart out and giving your all in races but still be finding that you just can't beat your personal best. It could be the case that you are actually over-training. As a result, your body is exhausted come race day, which prevents you from reaping the rewards of your efforts and reaching your full potential. To avoid over-training, take regular rest days. If you have done a particularly hard race, make this an extended rest period of a few days or a week.

In the build-up to a target race you should also ease back on your mileage so you have fresh legs on the day (known as tapering, see more on this in the marathon section in chapter five). For marathoners the taper period is three weeks, but if you are doing a half, 10k or 5k, taking it easy in the week preceding the race will suffice.

If you are disappointed with your training or race performances then consider other areas of your life that could be hindering your energy levels. It might be that you aren't getting enough sleep or aren't eating the right foods or drinking enough. If you have been having a stressful time you might also find your running suffers. If this is the case then don't be hard on yourself. Don't give up hope either – just because you haven't achieved a time you want yet, doesn't mean you never will. Also, remember that getting a PB when racing isn't the be-all and end-all.

WHEN 'COCKWOMBLES' TRY TO BRING YOU DOWN

'Cockwomble' is a word that has become popular in the RMR community. However, as comical as it sounds, when a member is suffering with one they rarely find it amusing. 'Cockwomble' refers to a partner who doesn't support their loved one's running endeavours. They might hinder their training by refusing to help with childcare, or undermine what they are trying to achieve, telling them they are a rubbish runner and so shouldn't bother.

Some might say you should leave such an unsupportive partner who doesn't allow you to flourish via running but the solution doesn't always have to be so drastic. Many cockwombles might just be a little bewildered by your newfound athleticism and may not understand why it is so important to you. Rather than argue or file for divorce, talk to one another. Explain why you are running and why you need, or would like, their help in order to do it. RMR's Tara Twyman says sometimes people can unintentionally exhibit cockwomble behaviour, and it can be caused by failure to communicate. She has the following advice: 'My husband is not a cockwomble. He's very supportive of my running in general, but sometimes he does make me feel guilty for being out training in the evenings and weekends – which is obviously when I have to do it because that's when he's home to look after our children. We just talk about it and usually reach a compromise! It's easy to say that partners should be supportive but it does work both ways. For us the key to keeping everyone happy is to communicate.'

If you are living with a cockwomble whose actions go beyond just being annoying – if they exhibit controlling behaviour over you by trying to prevent you running, or if their criticism becomes worrying and nasty – then do talk to someone and seek help, either from friends or family or a professional, such as a relationship counsellor.

Some RMR members have also extended the word to cover anyone in general who doesn't aid their running and seeks to criticise them and bring them down; the word 'frockwomble' is now often used to refer to female versions of a cockwomble. If you have been the victim of such negativity then don't let it get to you. Focus on why you love to run and all the benefits it's bringing you, and forget about the haters. Rest assured you will never be criticised or belittled as part of the RMR community. We promote kindness and are all about building women up, not bringing them down.

▶**Know when to take a break:** Sometimes when you discover a love of running it can become all-consuming. If you have deemed your partner to be a cockwomble because they're suddenly complaining that they never see you, then put yourselves in their shoes. They might just be feeling left out and upset because they miss spending time with you. Consider timing your runs so it doesn't impact on your time as a family. Or why not try to get them (and your children) to go running with you so you can be together while both getting active? If they don't or can't run, then involve them in other ways instead, such as by sharing your running aims with them and getting them to support you at races. Getting her partner more involved worked for RMR's Jennifer McLarnon. She said: 'Mine has always been supportive but being a wheelchair-user he can get a bit despondent that I'm off again for a run. Four months after I took up running we went for a run/push together and he loved it! He pushed and I ran, sprinting like a demon on the downhills to keep up with him. I think lots of cockwombles can redeem themselves – they just need to find out for themselves how awesome it is to run!'

RUNNING DURING PREGNANCY

Numerous studies have found that gentle exercise can be hugely beneficial to mums-to-be and their unborn babies. For the mums, it can lower the risk of gestational diabetes, prevent excess weight gain, alleviate nausea and help them deal with any anxiety surrounding parenting and the impending childbirth. Being fit and strong can also help in the final trimester and during labour.

Many women find running helps them feel happier and more energised so want to carry on with their hobby as their baby develops. However, if you haven't been a runner before becoming pregnant then it is not the time to start. Running also isn't recommended in the early stages of IVF treatment, or if you have any kind of complication in your pregnancy.

If you're used to running and have no pregnancy problems, then don't be afraid to do so in moderation. The NHS state exercise is 'not dangerous for your baby' and they recommend that mums-to-be continue with 'normal daily physical activity for as long as [they] feel comfortable'.

If you are running while expecting, always maintain a slow, steady pace where your heart rate doesn't get too high – you should still have breath enough to chat. It's imperative to avoid overheating, so don't wrap up too warm or go on a hot day.

Lots of RMR members have run while expecting and some have even taken part in races. One of them, Joanne Dennehy, has the following advice for expectant running mums: 'Get a bump support when you feel you need it – after around the eighteen-week point I was much more comfortable with it. Also do some strength training to avoid injury.' Vicki Rogerson adds that she found that 'running was a natural aid for morning sickness' but she switched to using an exercise bike at around 16 weeks as 'I needed a wee every mile!'

Cath Cook said she felt better for running when carrying her fourth child. She said: 'It's only a few kilometres every week but this is the first pregnancy that I continued running through, and I feel utterly fantastic for it. The worst part is the breathlessness but once the first kilometre is out of the way I don't notice it.' Meanwhile, Marina Parnell says that if you can still run while pregnant then make the most of it before life becomes more hectic. 'I wish I'd kept running when I was pregnant as it was hard to get going again after my son was born,' she said.

▶**Know when to take a break:** How much you can, and want, to run during your pregnancy will vary from mum to mum and could even change during each trimester. If you do feel up to it, don't run hard or for long distances. Always stop straight away if you feel any pain or discomfort. Don't force yourself to go out if you are feeling too tired, and don't try to stick to a strict schedule. Listen to your body and just run when you feel up to it. RMR member Jemma Hughes said she found transitioning to running while pregnant difficult at first but soon realised it was not the time to be trying to run at her best. She said: 'I was still running at thirty weeks. The hardest thing for me was mentally adjusting to the fact that it was okay to slow down. Initially I found it hard to accept as I've always been very target-driven in my running, but over time it's got easier. I learned to be proud that I was still running at all, rather than berating myself that I wasn't capable of running the same speeds and distances I was doing six months before.'

How long you carry on running is a personal choice and you shouldn't let anyone make you feel guilty about whether you are, or aren't, running when pregnant. Some mums stop when their bump starts to grow as they don't feel comfortable, and they switch to cycling, swimming or walking instead. Others are happy to keep jogging right up to their due date. Follow advice from your doctor and midwife as well as your own instincts on how you feel and what you are capable of. As they say, mum knows best!

When it comes to running after labour, it is not recommended to do so until at least six weeks after your baby's arrival. In creating and delivering a new life, your body has been through a huge change so you need to give yourself a chance to recover. In the case of a caesarean you will have to rest for longer, usually eight to twelve weeks, but seek advice from your doctors and midwives to be certain. When you've been given the green light to run again, resume gradually to avoid injury. You might find it best to redo the C25K or do some 'Jeffing' for a week or so before continuously running again. Your pelvic floor is likely to have been weakened so make sure you do strengthening exercises regularly. Your midwife or health visitor should have tips on this, and you can also see the section on stress incontinence (page 114) for further advice. For information on running and breastfeeding, see chapter four (page 129).

RUNNING WITH YOUR CHILDREN

It can be difficult to fit training in when you're a parent but there are lots of options to make it work which we outlined in chapter one, from using a running buggy to taking them to a junior parkrun. Of course, getting your child into running isn't just about making your own training more convenient. It's also about getting them fit and active, and helping them get into good habits that they will keep for life. Physical activity not only helps a child develop a strong, healthy body, but the mental benefits, such as improving concentration and alleviating anxiety, mean they do better at school and are more confident as well. Sport also helps them learn skills that will serve them well throughout life, such as determination, being a team player and how to handle winning and losing. According to the World Health Organization, 'physically active young people more readily adopt other healthy behaviours (e.g. avoidance of tobacco, alcohol and drug use) and demonstrate higher academic performance at school.'

It recommends children and young people aged 5–17 should accumulate at least 60 minutes of moderate- to vigorous-intensity physical activity a day.

Getting children interested in running can be a battle so make it fun for them. You could do relay races as a family, or turn a running route into a nature or treasure trail. If this doesn't appeal, you might find they prefer to run with those their own age, so see if your local athletics club caters for children – many allow youngsters to join from the age of eight upwards. Clubs often encourage them to participate in local races and give them the opportunity to try different disciplines as well as running, like the long jump. Being involved in such a group will mean your child's training can be overseen by expert coaches, and they can socialise with friends at the same time.

▶ **Know when to take a break:** If a child doesn't share your passion for running then don't force them to follow in your footsteps. You are setting them a wonderful example by being active but they don't have to run in order to get fit. Let them try lots of different sports and decide for themselves which they like best. The important thing is to help them find a form of exercise they love. That way, they will be much more likely to carry on with it into their adult life, reaping all the health benefits in the process.

If they do get into running, then don't encourage them to run long distances too soon. Under-11s are advised to race a maximum of 5k, under-14s 10k, and under-16s no more than a half marathon. Marathons are not advised until the age of 18 – as a result, many road races will specify a minimum age for entrants.

RUNNING WITH YOUR DOG

Your pet pooch could be your ideal running partner. Always full of enthusiasm and bounding with energy, their lust for exercise can rub off on you too. On days when you might not feel like going out for a run, they can provide motivation. Since you have to take them for a walk, why not run? Running with your dog can strengthen the bond between you both and give you some company.

Many of the habits you have with your own running regime should extend to your dog's – from not doing too much too soon to keeping them hydrated. If you're planning on getting a family pet and hope to be able to run with them too, do some research first to ensure you pick a breed suited to the sport. Border collies, huskies, spaniels, retrievers, pointers and Labradors are just some who are born to run, so there are plenty of options to choose from. But remember: dogs are for life, not just for running, so do consider first if you have the time to give a dog the care and company, as well as the exercise, they need before getting one.

If you do want to run with your dog, get them a harness so their lead can be attached behind their shoulders rather than to a collar. Not only will this allow them to breathe more easily when running, it will also give you greater control over the direction they move in. Elasticated leads are a good idea as they will prevent you getting jarred if your dog pulls or suddenly comes to a halt. Hands-free leads are also available, which you can attach to a belt around your waist.

While many dogs are trained to 'heel' and stick beside their owners when walking, it's better if your dog is slightly ahead to give you both more space to move when running. To begin with, you might find they are so overexcited about going out for a run they will speed off and drag you along behind (you are bound to pass someone who jokes 'who is taking whom for a run?'). But they'll soon settle into your pace when they have calmed down and have got used to running with you. If you can take them on a route where they can run safely off the lead, this will give you both the opportunity to go at your own pace.

It's worth teaching your dog a few basic commands to make running with them easier and safer. Go for short words in case you are out of breath, such as 'stop', 'wait' and 'go'.

You can race with your dog too. parkrun allows dogs on short leads to take part, while there are numerous events organised by groups such as CaniX.

▶ **Know when to take a break:** Just like us, dogs need to build up their fitness gradually so start them off with some run-walking until they are fit enough to run continuously. Puppies shouldn't start going on runs until they are at least eight months old, and for some larger breeds it might be 18 months until they are fully developed, so always check with their vet first. Never take them out on a very hot day – dogs don't sweat and instead cool down by panting, so they can easily become exhausted by the heat. Dogs can be so keen to run that they don't always know when to stop, so make sure yours has regular rest days and annual check-ups with the vet.

RUNNING AS YOU AGE

Women of all ages are welcome to join RMR, so as well as mothers we have grandmothers and great-grandmothers in the group. One of the great things about running is that age isn't a barrier. Numerous studies have found that being fit helps people look and feel younger as they get older, and keeps many age-related illnesses at bay. As we age, our muscle mass decreases and our metabolism slows down, so running can be hugely beneficial in terms of helping our bodies stay toned and strong and avoiding weight gain.

For women, starting or carrying on exercise is particularly valuable when going through the menopause. This usually occurs between the ages of 45 and 55 when the levels of oestrogen and other sex hormones fall, and periods peter out. Symptoms can include hot flushes, mood swings and night sweats, and it can also leave many women feeling lower in confidence. The hormonal changes can also lead to weight gain and increase the risk of developing weak bones (osteoporosis). Running can help immensely during this time. It helps keep the bones strong, aids sleep, burns calories and boosts self-esteem. Studies have found that women who exercise during the menopause have fewer symptoms and feel happier and more confident. This has certainly been the case for a number of RMR members, including Kirsty Rose. She said: 'Running has helped me cope with menopausal hot flushes and actually I don't suffer with them when I'm running regularly. It also helps me to keep my weight under control and alleviates the horrible menopause headaches and anxiety I get. I'm forty-nine and since I started running, I've done four half marathons and a couple of 10ks. I never dreamed I'd be able to do that at my age. Running has not only made me feel fitter than I have been for many years, but it's made me grow in confidence too. I now know I can do anything if I believe I can.'

Lesley Butlin had a similar experience: 'I started running at the age of forty-eight after losing a friend to cancer as I set myself a challenge to run the Race For Life 5k. At fifty, I did first my 10k and then at fifty-one my first half. I am now slimmer and my sleep during the menopause has improved, as well as my mental and emotional health. I generally feel less stressed, more confident and I'm loving life.'

If you haven't run before and you're in your fifties, sixties or beyond, it's not too late to start, as RMR member, Denise Taylor, discovered. She said: 'My "midlife crisis" at fifty took the form of losing four stone and taking up running. I have done several 5k and 10k races and I'm signed up for the Disneyland® Half Marathon Weekend in September, which I'm running with my nieces!'

Tina Copcutt, 59, is another member who took up running in her fifties, inspired by her active daughter. She said: 'I've joined a club and dropped from a size sixteen to eighteen to a size ten to twelve. It also helped with the menopause symptoms. Now I'm looking to do a longer run with more training, and even my husband has started running too.'

Meanwhile Carole MacFadyen ran a parkrun on her sixtieth birthday after taking up running nine months previously to support her son who also wanted to get fit. She said: 'He gave up but I got the running bug. I can now run eight miles and have signed up for two half marathons. I feel fitter, happier and a lot more confident than ever before in my life.'

Ali Dolphin agrees that running has helped her surpass the fitness of her youth. She said: 'I'm fifty-nine and took up running three years ago (after a brief spell in my late forties). I'm way fitter than I have ever been and am really proud that this non-sporty "old" lady has a parkrun PB of twenty-four minutes and one second, and 10k of forty-nine minutes and fifty-six seconds!'

If you want to follow in the footsteps of these inspirational ladies, begin by run-walking or following the C25K plan (see chapter two, page 56). Don't think that if you are menopausal you are beyond your peak either – recent research found that the menopause can actually make women fitter, as the reduction in oestrogen can improve the take-up of oxygen in the muscles.

As well as running, strengthening exercises such as pilates and weight-lifting will also help keep the bones strong into old age.

▶ **Know when to take a break:** It can take longer to recover from hard exercise as we age so it is important to be mindful and not expect to bounce back as quickly as you might have done in your youth. You might have to adapt your training by doing less mileage, or by taking more rest days than you did in the past. When it comes to avoiding injury the same rules apply to older generations as to the young — listen to your body, increase your training gradually and allow yourself adequate recovery after a strenuous workout.

RMR STORIES

'I found running empowering as I trained and raced whilst having chemotherapy': Nicky Lopez, 43, a mother and jewellery-maker from Liverpool, took up running when she was diagnosed with cancer and found that it saved her life in more ways than one.

Seven years ago I thought my world was coming to an end when I was diagnosed with cancer. In fact, a new stage of my life was beginning.

I was devastated to be told I had non-Hodgkin lymphoma, a form of cancer that develops in the lymphatic system, and I would need intensive chemotherapy to treat it. It was at this time I inexplicably decided to take up running. It was completely uncharacteristic. I had never picked up a pair of running shoes before and, having worked as cabin crew before becoming a teacher, I felt much more comfortable in high heels than trainers.

A Race For Life 5k was my first run. I kept seeing Cancer Research UK advertising the events to raise funds and it began to sink in those adverts were about me, so I decided to take part. It was a painful run that took nearly 50 minutes to complete owing to my not having done one bit of training. I thought that because I was skinny I would be naturally fit – how wrong could I be? Every single part of my body hurt. But I'm as proud of that finish time as any I've done since – prouder, maybe, because it was my first and I didn't let it be my last.

After that, things started to fall apart. Treatment began and failed, my initial positive prognosis became extremely bleak. With it, something changed in me – that's when I really became a runner, motivated by a desire to take back some control over what was happening to me. During chemo, my body seemed to belong to everyone else and I had to give myself over to drugs. But when I was running, I was the one deciding what to do with my own body. I was taking back control.

I signed up for a charity place at the Great North Run in 2011 and set myself on a path that would reshape my entire world. I trained and raced during my treatment, even though chemo can cause a number of problems that make exercise difficult. For example, I had trouble with balance, my sight was compromised and I became deaf in one ear. The drugs made the soles of my feet numb, which meant I couldn't tell when I'd rubbed blisters or sustained cuts; I had to check regularly, otherwise I'd get home to find my feet were shredded. Chemo also causes diarrhoea and weight gain from steroids. But I had grown to love running, and I wasn't going to stop. It was helping me in so many ways, particularly as chemo is so dehumanising. All your feminine qualities go – your hair, nails, you gain weight. I found running empowering as people don't care if you look feminine or not when you're running. They care that you look strong. I also love the physical and motivational side of it and the feeling of accomplishment.

It was also thanks to my newfound interest in the sport that I met my partner, Marc. He's become my running buddy, best friend, dad to my daughter Cleo and my comedy sidekick. Running is an intrinsic part of our lives and so we decided to run the 2013 London Marathon together in aid of the charity Macmillan Cancer Support. The charity had done so much for me, so I wanted to do something for them. They were fully supportive of my plans to run, even though I was still undergoing chemo. The training was a real struggle but with Marc by my side and the support of friends and family we completed the marathon. At the time I thought 'never again' but I have since run the London Marathon twice more! I've also run the Great Manchester Run, the Wirral 10k, the Santa Dash in Liverpool and the Great North Run another four times. In one Great North outing I ran a sub two-hour time, which I was delighted with. I felt it was then that I became a runner and not a girl with cancer.

I'm now in remission thanks to the prolonged chemotherapy, radiotherapy and countless surgeries from the incredible doctors, nurses and therapists who refused to give up on me. I have been lucky, and I will never stop being grateful. Running helped get me through those dark days and I am now a different person. It may sound strange but cancer was as much my saviour as my nemesis. It has made me look at the world differently, heightened my appreciation for my health and led me to take up running, which remains a huge part of my life. I joined RMR in 2015 and found it to be supportive, kind-hearted and just a lot of fun. It's like gaining a gang of awesome girlfriends cheering you on in your victories and raising you up in your tough times.

The support and generosity of spirit I discovered is something I'd like to pass on to other runners, so I now run a successful jewellery-making business, with pieces featuring inspirational quotes that are designed to give runners hope and support. I've also helped others by starting a running club, and I have written a book about my experience with cancer called *Recovery Run*, which I hope people find inspiring (don't let your kids read it though as it's full of bad words!).

I hope I can show people that barriers to running can be overcome. You might find, like me, that it changes your life.

CHAPTER FOUR:
EVERYTHING YOU WANTED TO KNOW
BUT WERE TOO EMBARRASSED TO ASK

One of the special things about the RMR community is that women can share personal and embarrassing issues they may not feel comfortable talking about to anyone in person. As we have a closed group this also provides a degree of privacy, so members can ask questions without their other Facebook friends and family reading them too. They can also rest assured that their problem will be responded to with support and kindness from their fellow RMR members. Here we have rounded up some of the most common problems experienced by female runners and some tips on how to prevent or tackle them.

STRESS INCONTINENCE

Stress incontinence is a major cause of embarrassment for many women and occurs when the muscles supporting the bladder and urethra (the pelvic floor) aren't strong enough. As a result, they can give way when pressure is applied, for example by sneezing and laughing, causing some urine to leak out.

Often it is associated with mothers – as their pelvic floors are sometimes weakened by childbirth – and older women, as they can lose some bladder control as a result of ageing. Menopausal women are also more likely to suffer stress incontinence due to a drop in the hormone oestrogen. But pelvic floor specialist, Jenni Russell (jennirussell.com), says that the problem is far more widespread than that. One in three women in the UK are estimated to suffer from stress incontinence. She says that it's important for women to be aware of their pelvic floor before they age or become mothers in order to prevent it becoming an issue. She says: 'Often women don't think about the pelvic floor until they have a child but there are many women who are not mothers [who are] suffering. From the minute we are born, every muscle in the body plays a role in our everyday function of life. We don't see those muscles so we don't consider them, but they have such an impact on our posture, sex life, digestion, the way we move and our confidence.'

Many women only become aware of a weakness when they start running, as the motion applies force through the pelvis every time the foot strikes the ground. It's something numerous RMR members have been unfortunate enough to experience. One of them is Rose Stride who admits: 'I once wet myself on a treadmill running in the gym. You win some, you lose some!' Meanwhile, Emma Donaldson confessed: 'I wet myself at my first 10k – good job there was a towel for finishing – much more useful than a medal!'

While these RMR members have been able to see the funny side, for others it can be highly embarrassing if it leaves an obvious wet patch on their shorts. The dampness can also cause chafing and irritation, and even lead to a urinary tract infection. Some women feel so ashamed and worried that it puts them off them running altogether. But Jenni Russell says that anyone can reverse the problem by taking the right steps, so they shouldn't let it ruin their confidence, lifestyle or running ambitions. Try the following:

▶ **Contract and elevate:** One of the most common ways to do a pelvic floor exercise is to sit on a chair with the knees slightly apart, then contract the muscles of the pelvic floor by first imagining you are trying to stop passing wind, and then trying to prevent having a wee. Russell says that, when doing this, it's not only important to contract but to elevate the muscles rather than just squeezing them. She says: 'Imagine you are drinking up through a straw or zipping up to your belly button. It's all about lifting the muscles up. Once you have done this, hold the position for five to ten seconds, lower and repeat.'

Women often struggle to identify the correct muscles to work in this position, so Russell suggests trying the move on all fours first while feeling the perineum, which is located between the vagina and the anus. Russell says: 'Place your fingers on the perineum. Inhale and allow the perineum to "bear down" on the fingers. Exhale as you contract and try to elevate your perineum away from your fingers.' Once you have practised this you will know which muscles you should be working, so you can then progress to doing it when standing or sitting in a chair, without the need to feel the perineum. If you are still struggling to establish which muscles to contract there are gadgets on sale that can help, such as an egg-shaped device from elvie.com which you can insert in your vagina and pair with your mobile phone so you can be sent information on whether you are doing the exercises properly. Once you have mastered the exercise, you can easily do it discreetly when sitting or standing throughout the day.

▶ **Improve your posture:** If you have poor posture, you are going to have a poor running gait so you need to address this by strengthening your core. Russell says it is vital to have a strong core when you're doing impact sports, such as running, as these muscles 'are a natural girdle, protecting the spine and stiffening the waist to support the internal organs, and [help] to minimise the natural pressure that builds up within your body from overloading your pelvic floor. Strengthening these muscles will give better support to your pelvic floor muscles, with the bonus of better tone and shape to your lower abdominals.' Russell recommends the following moves to strengthen the core:

▶ **The plank:** The plank involves lying face down and then balancing your weight on your toes and forearms with your back straight – your shoulders and back should not be rounded, your lower back should not dip excessively and your bottom should not be sticking up. Your head needs to be held in line with the body with eyes facing down to the floor (i.e. not with the head raised to look up, or hunched to look down at the feet). This is often the most recommended move to improve the core but Russell advises those with weak pelvic floor muscles to do an easier version until they have mastered the technique, otherwise they could make stress incontinence issues worse. She says: 'If you don't hold the position correctly, you will be putting more intra-abdominal pressure on your pelvic floor which will be counter-productive.'

For a less intense version, Russell suggests resting on knees placed 45 degrees behind the hips, with the toes still on the floor. Hold the alignment and elevate the pelvic floor muscles before lifting one knee to extend the leg, while the other knee is still touching the floor. Then lower the raised knee back to the floor and repeat with the opposite knee raised. Russell says that once you have mastered this, you are ready to lift both knees at the same time to hold the traditional plank position.

▶**Superman stance:** Russell highly recommends this move which she does every day. She says: 'When on all fours, raise the left arm out straight, then at the same time, lift your right leg off the floor and hold it straight so your raised arm and leg are in line. Hold the position for thirty seconds and then repeat with the right arm and left leg raised. I will hold this position before going for a run as it is a good way to encourage the body to be more stable and it makes you more aware of your posture.'

▶**The bridge:** Lie on your back with your knees bent and your feet flat on the floor, near to your bottom. Engage the glutes and the muscles just behind your belly button and then raise your bottom and hips off the floor. Russell adds that 'keeping the middle of the knee in line with the second toe makes the glutes work more effectively'. Hold the position, lower the bottom and repeat.

▶**Be consistent:** Get into the habit of regularly doing exercises to improve your pelvic floor. Russell points out: 'To see improvements, you need to do it consistently – just like you need to run more than once a week to improve your fitness. It doesn't mean you have to spend hours a day but if you can give it a bit of attention every day for a couple of minutes, then you will see an improvement.' You can download apps and get fitness trackers to remind and help you to do these exercises.

▶**Eat healthily:** Avoid processed foods high in saturated fats and sugars, as these can hinder your digestion and lead to a compacted colon. Russell warns: 'A compacted colon can weigh as much as 10 lb and that's pressing down on your pelvic floor.' She also advises avoiding dishes that can irritate the bladder such as spicy foods, tomatoes and cranberries. Instead, eat plenty of foods high in vitamin C – such as kiwis, oranges, peppers, kale and broccoli – as it is good for collagen formation and the lower urinary tract. She also recommends eating 'good fats' such as avocado, eggs, nuts and coconut oil.

▶**Go easy on caffeine and alcohol but drink plenty of water:** As caffeine and alcohol are both diuretics they will make you want to go to the toilet more, so excessive amounts are best avoided before running. However, don't avoid drinking altogether in order to prevent a full bladder as you need to be hydrated to help you run. Russell warns: 'Note that the biggest mistake to make is to avoid drinking water as this may dehydrate the muscles, which will have an adverse effect on strength and tone, and the ability to hold urine in, in the long term.'

If you're worried you might need to go when on a run, pick a route where you can pass public toilets, or don't be ashamed to nip behind a bush if running off-road. Just make sure you perfect your aim to avoid a mishap like RMR's Sara Black once experienced! She admits: 'At the start of my first marathon in Athens in 2010 I decided to hop over the barrier for a last-minute wee. I went to my heart's content only to realise that I hadn't spread my legs wide enough and had peed all over my right foot! It was soaked. Needless to say I ended up with an enormous blister (which I named Boris) and it had to be drained the following day by a pharmacist. I've not made that mistake since!'

To avoid such a situation when racing, arrive with extra time so you can use the toilet at the start (more often than not there will be long queues!). Most mass-participation races have portable loos on the course, so check this in advance. That way, you don't have to panic if you don't reach the front of the queue before the start, or if you have a last-minute need to go as you cross the line.

▶ **Get adequate sleep:** Russell says getting plenty of sleep is key to combating stress incontinence as it gives the body time to repair, restore and rebuild itself. She says: 'Allowing the body adequate and quality time to recover helps the pelvic floor to avoid muscle weakness and laxity.'

By following the tips above for a number of weeks, women should see an improvement in the strength of their pelvic floor. To spare your blushes in the meantime, try running with a pad or invest in some specialist kit. For example, EVB Sport have shorts with an integrated lining to hold a pad in place and are made with moisture-wicking material to keep you comfortable should a leak occur.

If you have an extreme case, don't be afraid to seek help from a specialist like Russell or your GP, as surgery can sometimes be an option. Remember that you are not alone in suffering so don't feel embarrassed about asking for treatment.

Russell is passionate about getting women to consider their pelvic floor health, so she has come up with this poem which she hopes will remind us all to look after those little muscles that can have a big impact on our confidence, sex life and running enjoyment.

> *My pelvic floor, something you cannot see,*
> *Can either reward or debilitate me.*
> *I can choose to ignore it and not value its role,*
> *and then under the knife I may just have to go.*
> *Or I can choose to acknowledge, condition and enjoy,*
> *gripping and lifting and running with joy.*
> *A little attention a few moments a day,*
> *and I can confidently, continently be on my way.*

RUNNER'S TROTS

Unfortunately, bladder weakness isn't the only toilet trouble runners have to deal with. Another problem is so prolific it has been given its own name – 'runner's trots'. This is when you can experience symptoms of diarrhoea whilst running and desperately need to relieve yourself. It can not only be painful, as it causes stomach cramps that can hinder your ability to keep running, but also super embarrassing if you experience flatulence, and distressing if a toilet isn't immediately available.

The exact cause of runner's trots isn't known but it is more likely to occur if you are long-distance running, due to the continuous jostling of the bowels. The nerves experienced in the build-up to racing can also exacerbate the problem.

Those with Irritable Bowel Syndrome (IBS) or food intolerances are more likely to suffer. Some theories suggest that, as blood is diverted to the muscles to aid movement, the digestive system is therefore neglected and problems occur, while others claim that dehydration could also be a factor. To avoid such a call of nature whilst running, try the following.

▶ **Avoid certain foods:** For many runners, the trots occur because of excessive consumption of high-fibre foods before running, such as wheat bran cereals and dried fruits. Other foods that could cause problems are beans, spicy, greasy or high-fat foods such as takeaways and dairy products. Avoid having too much of any of these the night before or within hours of a run. Discovering which foods trigger runner's trots can sometimes be a process of trial and error, and you could find that it's caused by a food intolerance that's unique to you. If you do experience it, remember what you ate beforehand so you can avoid eating it before running in the future.

▶ **Don't try eating anything new before a long run/race:** As outlined above, while certain foods are generally more likely to cause runner's trots, there might be something that you are particularly sensitive to but that your friend could eat and be fine. So the night before a race, stick to a tried and tested pre-run meal to avoid any nasty surprises. Save the fun of trying out new dishes for your celebratory post-run dinner!

▶ **Avoid eating a meal at least two hours before running:** Giving your body at least two hours between eating a meal and running will give you time to digest your food properly. In the case of a larger meal, allow at least three hours.

▶ **Stay hydrated:** If you are dehydrated, your digestive system will struggle to function optimally so you need to drink plenty of water, especially if it's a hot day and you're sweating profusely (read more on staying hydrated in chapter six, page 214).

▶ **Experiment with gels and energy drinks:** Many find that excessive consumption of energy gels and drinks can cause stomach upset. While some manufacturers recommend consuming them every 20 minutes, some people will find this too much for their digestive system to cope with. Again, it can be a process of trial and error to work out your optimum intake, and you might find that you respond better to some brands or kinds of energy supplements over others. For instance, while gels work for some people, others find jelly sweets preferable.

Never try a product for the first time on race day. Instead, experiment with new gels and drinks on your long training runs to see which ones work best for you, and always check the use by date as ones that have expired could also make you feel unwell. However, be aware you might not need to take them at all unless you are running a long distance. For shorter runs and races just stick to water (read more on energy drinks and gels in the carb-loading section in chapter six, page 211).

If you do experience runner's trots, then if you gotta go, you gotta go. Hopefully your training route or race course will pass a public toilet or portable loo you can get to quickly. If not, you may have to brave diving into a cafe or pub to ask if you can use their facilities. If you're running off-road then take cover behind the bushes and just hope you're not interrupted by any passing dog walkers or local wildlife! It can be embarrassing, but in these moments think of Paula Radcliffe who has never let toilet troubles hold her back. The whole world was watching when she had to stop to relieve herself on the side of the road during the 2005 London Marathon, but she said she had no regrets as it meant she was able to go on and win the race.

A number of RMR members who were caught out were mortified at the time, but have since managed to see the funny side. Among them is Jenna Sleeman who admits: 'I was out on a twelve-mile run. When I got to mile eight my stomach started churning. I quickly looked for a bush I could go behind. There was nothing, so I clambered up a hedge and across a ditch of brambles only to be met by a barbed wire fence. Luckily I made it safely to the other side just in time to go. Only after thinking "phew, I made it", I then spotted someone walking their dog. I pretty much high-jumped back over the fence, tearing my running leggings, and sped off home. Still no idea to this day if they saw me!'

Clare Matthews reveals that it's such a relief when you can go to the loo, you'll soon forget about any humiliation. She said: 'I was on a run along the sea front when I started getting stomach cramps, it was so bad I had to pause to breathe and clench. I knew there were toilets at the end of the beach but it was gone five o'clock and they were locked. Oh no! I started running toward the next beach, which was about half a mile away, doing a combination of run-walking and clenching. I looked to passers-by like I was in the Ministry of Funny Walks! Thankfully that toilet was open. I had such a spring in my step once I was done and was on way home with no more cramp – but I dread to think what would have happened if that toilet had been locked!'

PERIODS

The onset of a period every month can bring painful stomach cramps and make you feel highly emotional. You might be bloated due to water retention and feel like going for a run is the last thing you want to do. However, running can actually help; many find their tummy pains ease with gentle exercise, while the endorphin boost banishes their blues. It's easy to run in tampons and pads; with the latter, you may find ones with wings will be more secure as you move. However, the wings may chafe your inner thighs, so apply some anti-chafing gel between your legs before you go. Some women prefer to use menstrual cups that are inserted inside the vagina to catch drips. Such products recommended by RMR members include Mooncup, Femmecup and DivaCup. To prevent toxic shock syndrome, make sure you don't wear them for long periods of time or sleep with them in overnight.

Wash them thoroughly between uses and boil them regularly to kill off any bacteria.

Some find running in our skorts (running skirts) or a running dress preferable to running in shorts when it's that time of the month, as it means they don't have to feel self-conscious about any bulky sanitary pads being obvious. A tutu might not be a wise idea though, as Christina Walker has discovered! She said: 'I do long charity runs wearing a tutu and two years ago when I did the Great North Run it was my time of month. I can't use tampons and it was a hot day so I was tipping water over myself constantly. Needless to say, my sanitary towel expanded and I looked like I was wearing a nappy by the end of the run!'

While the onset of a period is usually more of a hindrance than an obstacle to running, it can be more problematic if it falls on a race day. There is no conclusive evidence that having a period can hugely impair performance, but every woman reacts differently. Some find being on their period has no effect on their running, but others – from elite athletes to recreational runners – say it puts them at a disadvantage both physically and mentally, and as a result they struggle to perform at their best. If you have been training hard for a big race and are expecting your period on the day, you could see your GP and ask if they can prescribe you a progesterone pill that will delay your bleed by a few days. However, just be aware that this could cause side effects that could also disrupt your ability to achieve a PB, if that's your goal.

If you aren't trying to conceive, you could also consider going on the contraceptive pill so that you have more control over your cycles and can time taking them to avoid race day menstruation. The contraceptive pill can also make periods lighter for those who suffer from heavy bleeding. However, if you don't want to take it there are alternatives. For instance, some RMR members recommend having a hormonal coil fitted to ease excessive flow. If you are suffering from this problem, speak to your GP about the options available to you.

If you're experiencing period pain before a run or race then never take anti-inflammatory drugs such as ibuprofen to deal with it, as they can dehydrate you and damage your kidneys. Take paracetamol instead. If you prefer natural remedies, try heating your tummy with a hot water bottle or some find the herbal remedy Agnus Castus beneficial. If you do feel in too much pain to run, then you might find other gentle exercise such as walking or pilates could help instead.

Foods high in magnesium can also help to ease cramps. This means eating leafy greens, beans, nuts, avocados and – hooray! – dark chocolate. Another reason to up your consumption of leafy greens during your time of the month is because they're high in iron. The loss of blood can deplete your iron levels and make you feel weak, so eating plenty of foods high in this mineral can help. Broccoli, beef, nuts and pumpkin seeds are also high in iron so are worth including in your diet too. If your iron levels are particularly low, leaving you constantly feeling lethargic and light-headed, you might need to take an additional iron supplement such as a vitamin tablet.

INFERTILITY

For some runners, periods aren't an inconvenience because they simply aren't having them. Not only is this bad news if you want to have a baby, but failing to have a regular bleed when you should be having one can be detrimental to your womb and bone health, so always see your GP if you have gone more than six months without having a period (unless you're pregnant or breastfeeding).

A lack of menstruation is known as amenorrhoea. For some women this occurs due to a medical condition, but it can also be prevalent in runners with low body fat who are training particularly hard. If they're not eating enough nutrients to fuel their workouts, their periods can cease or become irregular, both because their body feels under stress, and because any food that is taken on board is directed to where it is needed to aid running rather than reproduction. This is not only an issue for those wanting to conceive, but it can also lead to a number of other serious health complications, for instance, osteoporosis, which makes you much more likely to suffer from a running injury such as a stress fracture. If you suspect you have amenorrhoea because you've been pushing yourself too hard then cut back on your training. Do less mileage, fewer hard interval sessions and try to increase your body fat. This doesn't mean you have to pig out on unhealthy foods. Instead, fill up on good fats and nutritious dishes that will nourish and sustain your body. If your periods don't return and you are concerned about any other associated health complications, speak to your doctor.

For around one in five women in the UK, a lack of or irregular periods is due to a condition called polycystic ovary syndrome (PCOS). In their case, exercise, such as running, is a recommended activity to ease the symptoms and maintain a healthy weight because it helps to manage their abnormal insulin levels. If you have PCOS and want to have a baby, then visit your GP to discuss your options. They will be able to advise you on lifestyle changes or may prescribe drugs that could help.

If you are having regular periods but are still struggling to conceive, then also see your GP to have yourself and your partner tested to investigate what the problem may be. Running could be beneficial to you during this time as it will help you maintain a healthy body, and relieve any stress and anxiety you might be experiencing as a result of failing to have a baby. If your pregnancy quest leads to you taking fertility drugs and having IVF, then do check with your doctor about how much exercise it's safe to do at this time.

Many women will find that there's no reason for them to stop running when trying for a baby – they just need to remember to save plenty of energy for the bedroom!

BREASTFEEDING

If you choose (and are able) to breastfeed your baby, this doesn't mean you have to compromise your exercise regime when you are able to resume running after childbirth. If you feel embarrassed about the possibility of leakage showing on your running top then either feed your little one or express milk before you go to make this less likely to happen. It will also make your boobs lighter, making running more comfortable. Wearing breast pads can also help if you fear leaking and they can prevent your nipples chafing and getting sore. You could also try applying anti-chafing gel to your nipples before you go as they are likely to already be cracked and sensitive from breastfeeding. Double check that it's okay to use the product while breastfeeding first, and wash it off before feeding your child again. Some RMR members also swear by the old wives' tale of putting cabbage leaves inside their bra to alleviate pain and swelling.

As your breasts get bigger and heavier when feeding, you will probably find you need to go one or two sizes up in your sports bra. Get yourself measured if you're not sure about your size. Some find doubling up with a bra and a crop top is useful both for support and hiding potential leaks.

There is no evidence to prove that running while breastfeeding is detrimental for the health and growth of your baby. Moderate exercise will not affect your supply or the nutrients your child gets from your milk. Some studies have found that the amount of lactic acid in the supply increases if mothers exercise 'to exhaustion' when breastfeeding, but most won't have the energy or inclination to do this whilst also caring for a new baby. The Australian Breastfeeding Association sum up worldwide research on their website where they state: 'There is no evidence to suggest that breastmilk with increased lactic acid levels harms a baby in any way.' They also say there is no evidence that breastfeeding can 'cause, maintain or worsen' weak pelvis conditions that may have been caused by labour, and conclude that 'provided the mother is comfortable, breastfeeding is not a reason why a mother has to avoid any form of exercise.'

If you are exercising when breastfeeding, make sure you keep your energy levels up by eating healthy meals and snacks and drinking plenty of water to stay hydrated. Try expressing and storing milk so someone else can feed your baby if your only window to go is when they are hungry. If you decide to take them out with you in a running buggy when they are old enough (see page 30 for more information on this), don't be embarrassed to stop and feed them mid-run if you have to. Pack a shawl into the buggy so you can use it to cover your chest if you want to be more discreet.

'WOBBLY BITS'

At RMR, we celebrate women of all shapes and certainly don't believe you have to be a certain size in order to run. Never feel that you shouldn't run or join a club because of your size – it is an activity for all. However, if you are worried about your weight and feel you could improve your health and happiness by losing a few pounds, then start with the Couch To 5k plan outlined in chapter two (page 56).

The RMR page is full of inspiring before and after pictures showing how some members have experienced amazing body transformations after taking up running. Many of them started in the first place because weight-loss was their goal but kept it up because they found a love for the sport. This was the case for Hannah Jones, who said: 'I started to run to lose weight but discovered so much more. It has given me a newfound confidence in myself, I've made some amazing friends and feel valued. So now I run because it makes me feel good in lots of ways.' Vicki McBride had a similar experience. She said: 'I started running as an aid to maintain weight that I had lost from just walking for exercise, but then I found that – shock of all shocks – I actually enjoyed it. I was forty-three and hadn't run since school, and I couldn't run for two whole minutes before collapsing, but I graduated the C25K app and did my first parkrun to celebrate. My aim was to just run 5k, but since then I have done a few 10k races, a half marathon and I have entered the Brighton Marathon. I'll never break any records but running has given me such a sense of achievement in myself and pride that I can, and will, do what I put my mind to. I now run for the running, and the weight maintenance is just an added bonus.'

If losing weight is your reason to run but you find you're not having as much success as you would like, then consider tweaking your diet too. Beware of consuming too many sugary energy drinks during and after your run, and try not to get into the habit of rewarding yourself with a naughty food treat after every time you've exercised. However, we wouldn't recommend following a strict deprivation diet or cutting out treats altogether; you need carbs and sugar to fuel some of your runs and to eat enough to aid your recovery afterwards. Read more on running and nutrition in chapter six (page 201).

If you have only been running at an easy to steady pace you might find that you can lose more weight if you start doing some faster-paced runs, such as fartleks or interval sessions, as these raise your heart rate and lead to you burning more calories. We'd also recommend doing regular strength and conditioning exercises such as squats and core stability, not for aesthetic purposes, but to give you a stronger body that is less likely to get injured. Don't get hung up about the number on the scales. Muscle is denser than fat, so as you get fitter and develop a more toned physique you may find that your overall weight isn't that different.

Please remember that life is too short to get paranoid about what our bodies look like, and most of us don't have time to train as hard as an Olympian! We all do the best we can with the time we've got, and that's something to feel proud of. Rather than weight-loss, focus on training for the joy of running and the increased fitness it brings you, and you'll love your body – wobbly bits and all – because of the incredible feats it can help you achieve.

CHAFING, BLISTERS AND LOST TOENAILS

Clothes and body parts rubbing when you run can often cause chafing, with sweat making the problem worse. Not only can this cause some unsightly marks on your skin, but it can be terribly painful. In extreme cases, such as in long-distance races, it can even cause nipples to bleed (although usually this is more of an issue for male runners than females, since their nipples can protrude more, and they don't run in sports bras which have a softer lining than a T-shirt or a vest).

To prevent your skin rubbing, get an anti-chafing gel and apply it anywhere you think your kit might rub, such as under your sports bra, under your arms if you're wearing a vest or around your groin if you are wearing shorts with an inner lining. Vaseline and Tiger Balm are cheap options, while some RMR members also swear by Body Glide. If you do end up with red, raw skin, make sure you moisturise to ease the pain and avoid wearing the garment that caused the problem until your skin has healed.

Another uncomfortable result of chafing is blisters, so don't forget to apply the gel around your feet and ankles before a long run. If you have correctly-fitting trainers and wear running-specific socks, you are also less likely to suffer. If you do get a blister then try to resist the urge to pop it. The layer of water has been formed to cushion and protect the skin underneath while it heals, so popping it can delay the process and risk infection. The liquid will be reabsorbed by the skin in a few days. In the meantime, you could wear a plaster to stop it being irritated.

While we're discussing foot health, toenails can also become casualties on long runs if you don't take necessary precautions. Make sure your trainers aren't too tight and that you have plenty of room around the toes. If your toes press into the front of your shoe when you stand in them then you need a larger size. If they seem to have enough space when you're standing, but you then find your foot slides forward as you run, causing the toes to rub the front of the shoe, then you might also need a bigger size, a narrower fit, or to tie your laces more firmly. Another essential way to prevent losing any toenails is to always keep them cut short.

RUNNING COMMANDO

To avoid chafing around the groin and inner thighs, the solution for some RMR members is to go commando! Many attest that running around the streets without knickers when no one else is any the wiser makes them feel liberated and just a little bit illicit. Just make sure the elastic on your shorts or leggings is tight enough to avoid them falling down and giving away your secret! Penny Nash admits that this happened to her and, even though she hadn't gone commando, she has still never lived it down. She said: 'I was running a 5k and, at the start, the elastic went in my leggings. I had to keep pulling them up, but I was wearing a red thong underneath and one time I grabbed my thong by mistake. This gave me a wedgie as well as mooning the runners behind! At that point also I went past the photographer who took a photo and burst out laughing. Luckily he was a friend of mine, but another of the runners I mooned was a governor at the school I work at!'

RMR MEMBERS SHARE THEIR EMBARRASSING STORIES AND HOW THEY SAW THE FUNNY SIDE

From wardrobe malfunctions to toilet troubles, mortifying situations can happen to us all when running. Here, RMR members reveal incidents which have left them feeling very red-faced – but which they can laugh about now!

Beware of wayward sports bras...

> *'I had a wardrobe malfunction during a half marathon when my sports bra untied about three miles in. I was running on my own and no one I knew was close-by so I had no option but to ask a complete stranger who was spectating to do it up again. I was so embarrassed. I looked for the kindest-looking female to help, as running with an undone bra is not possible for a larger-breasted woman! I have never lived that one down!'*
> Leah Hill

> *'I ran for five miles with my boobs flopping about after they fell out of my sports bra. No wonder everyone was beeping and encouraging me on!'*
> Rachel Whitfield

'I was road-testing a new zip-front, racer-back sports bra under a baggy vest and doing some impressive intervals between the lamp posts in the local park when the zip came undone and my right boob "bounced" out! It happened right in front of a male dog walker! I'm not sure who was more red-faced as I smiled, waved and tucked the wayward boob back in and he stuttered, "Good morning!"
Priceless moment!'

Helen Mitchell

Caught out by runner's trots...

'I ran thirteen miles with a friend then I carried on by myself. Just after I left her, I felt a huge shift in my stomach. I had to dive over a wall where there was an underpass. Let's just say I had to stop and drop. It was instant. Broad daylight, no bushes! Anyone could have walked by. It was an experience I will never forget. I was mortified at the time but can laugh about it now.'

Paula Cowley

Watch where you squat…

'I needed the loo and managed to find a bush to squat behind quickly – straight onto thorns! In a rush to pull my leggings up, I managed to tuck some thorny branches into my knickers, it took me five miles to get them out of my pants!'

Emily Calcutt

'I once went behind a tree and I was so desperate that I didn't see that I had just sat on stinging nettles. I couldn't sit down for a week!'

Louise Maule

Singing shame…

'I remember someone telling me that the best fat-burning happens when you can talk and run, so I used to sing along to my music. I was on an early-morning run at about six thirty a.m. and I decided to sing along to a song with a lyric about preferring someone without their clothes on! I turned a corner and faced three businessmen on their way to the train station who found it very funny! I have never sung while running since!'

Amanda Smith

Always watch where you are going...

'I ran on holiday and fell down a manhole in Greece! It was
so deep I had to raise my arms to haul myself out!'
Louise Milward-Lawson

'I broke my ankle in two places at the London Marathon –
and I wasn't even running it that year! I toppled over
a parking cone and wasn't at the end to see my
best friend finishing.'
Alison Dale

When beauty treatments go wrong...

'I went to get my eyebrows tinted and had planned to run
afterwards. Halfway through my run I noticed people kept
staring as they drove past. Turns out the beautician hadn't
wiped all the black dye out of my brows and my sweat had
made it run all down my face! I looked like a zombie!'
Charlie Freeman

Mishaps with an audience…

'I was running on my normal Thursday route at Virginia Waters when I went across the polo fields. Halfway across, the irrigation system came on and I was totally drenched. I thought nobody saw but as I turned around and dried my eyes, I saw the entire polo team in absolute fits of laughter!'
(another) Amanda Smith

'I was running along the canal towpath feeling very smug, singing to my heart's content when I caught my toe on something. I fell flat on my face. I got up super quickly to check that no one had seen only to find a barge passing with six teenagers all with their phones laughing – YouTube alert!'
Tracey Francis

Treadmill trips…

'I fell off the treadmill at the gym. After placing one foot on the plastic bit at the side that doesn't move, I sort of did the splits and then face planted. Luckily, all I hurt was my pride!'
Amie Day

'I was at a circuits session at the gym. I followed the person in front onto the next exercise – which happened to be on the treadmill – and they had left the machine running! I hopped on and was promptly chucked off the end!'

Emma Poulter

Laughter isn't always the best medicine…

'My husband had suggested a comedy podcast to listen to while running, I decided to use it during a dreaded hill session to spur me on – I laughed so hard I full-on weed myself.'

Tracy Lawrence

Thunder pants…

'I was running on a beautiful summer evening. Every step I took I gave out the loudest farts ever – they echoed around the fields. I then ran past two people arguing over whether they really had heard thunder!'

Penny Nash

CHAPTER FIVE:
RACE MUMMY RACE!

WHY RACE AND HOW TO GET INVOLVED?

You don't have to join in any races in order to be a runner, but for many they are one of the most enjoyable aspects of the sport. Targeting a race can be a great way to stay motivated to train, either by encouraging you to get the miles in if you are preparing for a long-distance event, or by making you train harder so you can go faster to achieve a PB time.

Being part of a race – particularly mass-participation ones, like those in the Great Run Series and big-city marathons – is a magical experience. There will be a carnival atmosphere with bands on the route, hordes of crowds cheering you on, and you'll be surrounded by hundreds of other like-minded runners. During a race, your emotions can run the gamut from terrible nerves at the start, to low points where your legs will tire and you feel you can't carry on, to elation at seeing the sign for the finish, followed by triumph at crossing the line. We can bet that no matter how difficult you found it was to get there, you'll think 'when can I do this again?' shortly after.

As well as giving you a feel-good buzz, a cherry on top of finishing a race is a prize you can show off with pride, such as a shiny medal or a commemorative T-shirt. Many give out goody bags to finishers as well, and if you're speedy you could also win a prize in your age category.

Taking part in your first race can be extremely nerve-racking. If you're worried, try joining in a few parkruns first (see more on parkrun on page 145). They're not technically races but 'timed runs', so they can build up your confidence by giving you experience of many elements of a race – a mass start, camaraderie with other participants and the euphoria of crossing the finish line – without any pressure to be competitive or to finish in a certain time.

Once you've decided to give racing a go, you'll find there are a multitude to choose from, both in the UK and around the world. Check out the events listings in running magazines, on websites such as runbritain.com and keep your eyes peeled for posters advertising races in your area. Joining a club will also give you the opportunity to get involved; if your club takes part in certain leagues, they may even pay for your entry into certain races as a perk of membership. This is also a wonderful way to experience some team spirit as you'll have your fellow club mates there to support you and, in these kinds of races, your performance – no matter how fast or slow – often contributes to the overall team score.

Race distances and terrain vary widely. The traditional distances raced are 5k, 5 miles, 10k, 10 miles, half marathon (13.1 miles) and marathon (26.2 miles). Anything beyond 26.2 miles is classed as an ultramarathon. Races can be held on roads, through woodlands and countryside (known as off-road, cross country or trail running) or on mountains (known as fell running). Track races come under the athletics umbrella and range in distances from 100 m to 10,000 m. Some ultras are also held round (and round and round) tracks. Anywhere and everywhere could be a race venue as long as there's someone able to organise it safely and people willing to take part. More obscure events have been held up skyscrapers (known as tower running), round multi-storey car parks, in deserts and in the jungle. The choice is yours regarding how much you want to challenge yourself in terms of distance and conditions – but keep in mind that you'll always need the time to train to ensure success, so consider what's feasible for you before signing up. Many get caught up in 'marathon fever' because they are often the most publicised events, but they also require a lot of training. You're just as much of a runner whether you race 5k or 26.2 miles (or if you don't race at all) so don't feel obliged to run a marathon if it isn't currently right for your level of fitness or life commitments.

If you're worried about being at the back of a race then take a look at the results from previous years to see the finishing times of the last runners. It's also advisable to double check to see if there is a cut-off time for participants. Not all races have them but some have to do so for safety reasons, so don't take it personally if you find you're not going to be fast enough to take part. It might be that the organisers can't get enough marshals to monitor the course for a lengthy period, or there may be a limit to how long the roads used can be closed to traffic. There are plenty of races to cater to all paces, so there will be many more options open to you. Check out recommendations from RMR members over the following pages.

RMR MEMBERS REVEAL THEIR FAVOURITE UK 5Ks

Here are details on 5k events staged across the UK which get a big thumbs up from our members.

PARKRUN

parkrun has grown from a small group of runners meeting for a Saturday morning 5k run in the park to a worldwide phenomenon. At the time of writing, there are 478 parkruns taking place every Saturday morning, mostly in the UK with a handful of others in countries including Denmark and Australia. They are so prolific, with the number of events growing every week, that there's bound to be one near you. If not, why not consider setting one up in your local park? Find out more on how to do this in chapter seven, page 232.

We're talking about parkrun here in our race chapter but they are actually timed 5ks – not races – so there is no pressure to finish fast and you don't have to be competitive. There will be some speedy runners at the front, and you can treat it as an opportunity to run as fast as you can, but it's equally fine to run at a leisurely pace whilst chatting to a friend.

Many RMR members have confessed to being fearful of attending parkrun for the first time as they believed they weren't 'good' enough. One of them was Sarah Gibb, who said: 'I was reluctant to parkrun at first as I thought it was just for fit, experienced runners – even though I was told that people of all shapes, sizes, fitness levels and ages go and that they all celebrate each other's success at whatever stage of their running "journey" they are on. I guess I was the world's biggest sceptic and had a bad case of low self-esteem and confidence. I finally plucked up the courage to go after a friend suggested we go together. Registering online was easy. The sense of community was awesome. I loved waiting to find out the time that I managed to achieve, and now I always look forward to the next parkrun so that I can try to improve my time (although time really doesn't matter, as the overriding message of parkrun is to get out and get moving – slow or fast – with a friendly, like-minded group of people). parkrun has enabled me to believe in myself and encouraged me to follow a healthy lifestyle. I will be fifty next year and can't believe that in my forty-ninth year I have discovered a hobby that I really enjoy to do. I plan to keep going as long as I am able to. I also love that I am inspiring my thirteen-year-old daughter and showing her the importance of lifelong exercise.'

As Sarah, and many other RMR members have discovered, when it comes to parkrun, it really is the taking part that counts. You can walk if you need to and you'll be surrounded by people of all ages and paces – from those running with dogs, to parents pushing buggies, to those joining in with their children. It's also impossible to come last, as a parkrun volunteer always walks at the back of the field and is recorded as the final finisher.

We are huge fans of parkrun at RMR as it is such a fun, inclusive event. There's a real community spirit around it. Some stage special events, such as inviting participants to run in fancy dress at Halloween and Christmas, and meeting up with your fellow runners for breakfast at a nearby cafe afterwards is encouraged. Even better, it's completely free! All you have to do is register at www.parkrun.org.uk and print off a personal barcode which you should take along with you on the day (and every time you take part). This barcode will be scanned at the end, along with a finishing token you will be given when you cross the line, so you can find out your time. You need to take your barcode along with you each time you take part if you want your time to be recorded. The parkrun website keeps a record of all the occasions your barcode has been scanned so it's an excellent way to track your progress and to work towards getting an exclusive 'milestone' T-shirt when you have notched up 10, 50, 100 or even 250 parkruns.

The event is always looking for volunteers to help stage and marshal the events too, so it's a good way to stay connected to the running community if you're unable to run, (through injury, for example), and to give something back. Read more about 'paying it forward' this way in chapter seven, page 231.

parkrun is such an enjoyable, social way to keep your running on track, we are certain you will love it, and you're bound to bump into another RMR member there! Regulars include Liz Arnold who says: 'I have done over eighty. I go religiously and often join in with my running buggy. parkrun is so inclusive – there is a role for everyone and no one is out-of-place. My favourite thing is that the whole family can take part, and it's a fab start to the weekend.' Mandi Leech agrees. She says: 'I love parkrun, it's so friendly and welcoming. My hubby and I take it in turns to buggyrun and even my daughters aged eight and twelve have started coming too. I never thought my daughter would run yet she is, because of parkrun, and she loves it.' Henrietta Green adds: 'I can honestly say that parkrun has changed my life and our life as a family. Now, we wouldn't start the weekend any other way.' For more information visit parkrun.org.uk

CANCER RESEARCH UK'S RACE FOR LIFE SERIES

RMR have always been huge fans of this women-only race series. Organised to support the work of the charity Cancer Research UK, it's a fun run with a serious aim – money raised via sponsorship goes towards research into fighting the disease.

There are 5k runs in parks across the UK over the spring and summer. It's perfect for those who are new to racing and looking to build up their confidence, and those who want to join in a fun, friendly race. Participants are encouraged to wear pink and all abilities are welcome – you can run, walk or jog, go solo or team up with friends.

Such has been the popularity of the 5k events that Cancer Research UK now also organise 10ks and obstacle course races called Pretty Muddy, where you get just that. More recently, they have also started doing half and full marathons. For more information, visit raceforlife. cancerresearchuk.org.

RMR STORIES

'Race For Life started my love affair with running': RMR creator and founder, Leanne Davies, reveals why she loves Cancer Research UK's Race For Life series.

Race For Life was my first ever race ten years ago. I can still remember how it felt. I was sick with nerves and worried that I would make a fool of myself and that people would stare at me. How wrong could I have been? The race was amazing, everyone was smiling, people held hands, runners wore messages on their backs to celebrate or commemorate their loved ones, spectators clapped and smiled – how could I not be touched by this? I was on a complete high, I ran all the way round and even picked up my pace over the finish line – a complete success!

That day changed me, both as a runner and a person. It gave me a newfound confidence, and I knew that this was just the beginning of a new me and my long-term love affair with running. I can only thank Race For Life for this. Since then, I have competed in many more of the 5ks and I had such a fun time doing a Pretty Muddy event along with a group of other RMRs – we laughed the entire way round.

I was honoured in 2016 when RMR were invited to be one of Race For Life's official supporters. I never dreamed when I set up a small Facebook group of three runners that I would eventually be working with a charity I care so deeply about, and on this kind of scale. I feel that together we are a real force for good. Our collaboration is one of my proudest achievements with RMR. I hope many more women will discover the joy of running and racing via Race For Life like I did, while helping towards one day finding a cure for cancer.

THE COLOUR RUN

The Colour Run, started in 2011, is dubbed 'the happiest 5k on the planet'. Participants are given white T-shirts to run in and are showered with paint powder as they make their way around the course. The run is not timed and isn't competitive – it's just about getting round, whether you walk, run, skip or dance, while having fun in a riot of colour. The events are organised around the world by a for-profit event management company, with a number taking place in UK cities including Manchester, London and Brighton over the summer months. Children can take part too and the party continues after the run with a music festival.

In chapter two, RMR member, Hannah Hiscock, revealed how she loved taking part in The Colour Run, which she targeted at the end of a C25K plan. Kate Morgan is another fan of the series. She says: 'Colour Runs are the best two runs I've done, hands down. Seeing my kids, my best mates and their kids covered head-to-toe in rainbow colours, together with huge smiles, was heart-warming.'

Meanwhile, Noreen Groves said she loved taking part in The Colour Run with her daughter. She explained: 'It can be a nightmare to get my teenage daughter to exercise. However, she loved taking part in The Colour Run and needed no persuasion to get involved! We both loved it and at the end I had a teenager covered head-to-foot in various colours and smiling from ear to ear!'

For more information, visit www.thecolorrun.co.uk (note the U.S. spelling for the website).

BIG FUN RUN

Big Fun Run events are held in scenic locations in Scotland and England between July and October. Raising money for charity by taking part is encouraged, as is running with your whole family. Children under five can take part for free, and you can join in while pushing a running buggy. It is not timed and not competitive, as their website states: 'This isn't about Olympic level athletes charging about in record times, it's about mums with prams, dads with toddlers, groups running together, fancy dress and a fantastic fun mix.'

RMR's Rachel Finsbury is one of our members who recommends it. She says: 'The Big Fun Run is a great way to run your first 5k in a non-pressured way whilst still getting some running bling and raising some money for your chosen cause.'

To find out more, visit www.bigfunrun.com.

OTHER 5Ks TO LOOK OUT FOR

If you are keen to do a fun, 5k run, then any of the above events would suit you perfectly. Also, look out for fun runs held as part of big city marathons and half marathons. A shorter run will often be held the day or morning before the main event to create a fun festival of running.

There are also other runs organised similar to The Colour Run, where you can be splattered with paint, while 'Santa runs' are popular at Christmas time, in which participants dress up as Father Christmas. These are often arranged by charities so look out for one near you during the festive season.

If you are looking for a more competitive 5k and are keen to run a PB time, then search the race directory at www.runbritain.com to find one near you. Your local running club might also give members the opportunity to take part in 5k races as part of road race leagues they may compete in.

RMR MEMBERS REVEAL THEIR FAVOURITE UK 10Ks

We asked RMR members to nominate their favourite 10ks races around the UK and here are their top choices, divided by region.

SOUTH OF ENGLAND

▶**London Winter Run:** Dozens voted for this 10k in the capital, including Rebecca Howells who said she enjoyed it because it had 'a great atmosphere, [was] well organised, not terribly expensive and on closed roads. It's a great way to get the experience of running in central London without committing to the marathon, and it's topped off with pretty bling.'

▶**London 10,000:** This is another capital run given the thumbs up, because it's flat and passes many famous landmarks. Fans include Jo Webb, who said: 'Brilliantly organised. Running the closed roads of central London and seeing all the sights was fantastic.'

▶**Great Newham Run:** RMR members love this event, organised by the Great Run Company, because it finishes on the track in the London 2012 Olympic Stadium. Patricia Mitchell adds that it makes a good family day out, as spectators can explore the Olympic Park and get reduced entry to The ArcelorMittal Orbit, the UK's largest sculpture which is also an observation tower and a slide!

▶ **GEAR 10k Kings Lynn:** This is another race that's hugely popular with RMR members. Julie Jardine said that it's because it's 'a well-organised event in a beautiful town. The route goes around the river, through the park and town. It's quite flat with enormous support from community.' Tamara Cook agrees: 'Flat route, nice medal, great goody bag, well organised and loads of support from the locals – great for a PB.'

▶ **Stubbington 10k:** This race in a Hampshire village picked up a number of votes. Sophia Wheeler said: 'This was my first race, and the friendliness and great organisation spoiled me for any other.'

▶ **Windsor Women's 10k:** Many recommended this race, with Cathy Owen saying that this is thanks to 'the awesome final mile down the long walk with the castle right in front of you.'

▶ **Bournemouth Marathon Festival 10k:** This beachfront race has a number of fans including Paula Smith, who says it's 'really well organised with a fab atmosphere, and has great medals and goody bags.'

▶ **Bath Two Tunnels:** This is a favourite for its unusual setting. 'Two-and-a-half miles is underground!' describes Lucy Pitman.

▶ **Osterley 10k:** There were lots of nominations for this race in a National Trust owned estate. Marina Parnell said: 'It was well organised and a fab place to run.'

▶**Eastleigh 10k:** Another popular one with those living near the South coast, this race is described by Joanna Price as 'flat, fast and very well supported'.

Others highly rated were Run Norwich, Ipswich Twilight 10k and Dash In The Dark, Buckinghamshire.

NORTH OF ENGLAND

▶**Mad Dog:** RMR members voted in droves to say that this event in Southport, Merseyside was their favourite. Georgina Walker reveals why: 'Best goody bag around, the pens are dog themed and you howl to start the race! It always raises loads of money for charity too.' Sharon Barrett agrees, saying that the event is 'all-round fantastic', while Michelle Copeland says it has the 'best 10k atmosphere ever and an awesome goody bag!'

▶**Market Drayton 10k:** This is another hugely popular race with our members, many of whom love the unusual finishing gifts! Fiona Wright says: 'There's a great atmosphere and an awesome goody bag including things like yoghurts, pork pies and a gingerbread man.' Becki Corbett agrees, saying it has 'the best goody bag ever.'

▶**Langdale Christmas Pudding 10k:** This is another firm favourite ahead of the festive season thanks to the prizes for finishers. 'No medal – you get a full-size Christmas pudding! Perfect recovery food,' says Charlie Westney. Annabel Westney adds: 'As well as the full-size Christmas pudding at the end, the views of the fells are spectacular and the route isn't too hilly.'

▶**Lincoln 10k**: Katie Griffiths is among those who recommend this run because it's 'a good route, well organised and there's fantastic support on the course.' Sarah Angela Bentley adds that she loves the 'great T-shirt, the lovely medal and scenic finish.'

▶**North Tyneside 10k:** There are lots of fans of this race held on Easter Sunday. Marie Race says it's so popular because it has 'beautiful views, great support and it's a great way to justify an Easter egg!'

▶**Great Grimsby 10k:** This has been recommended by numerous members because you can take the whole family along for a day out. Katherine Simmons says: 'It's well organised, there's plenty of entertainment on the route plus a beautiful park finish with a family festival.'

Also highly rated are the Great Manchester 10k, Scarborough 10k, Wigan 10k and the Beverley 10k.

MIDLANDS
▶**Great Birmingham 10k:** This is another of the races in the Great Run series. Emma Gerrard said: 'It's by far my favourite as there were brilliant crowds, a fab medal and I loved the T-shirt. I would definitely do it again.'

▶ **Two Castles 10k:** Run between Warwick and Kenilworth castles, this is favoured by a number of members including Karen Hall, who says: 'It's a bit hilly but there's fab support from the locals.'

▶ **Worcester 10k:** Lots of members recommend this run by the River Severn because it is 'flat and fast and really well organised,' according to Sussanne Chambers. She adds that there are 'great goody bags, medals and T-shirts.'

Also highly rated are the Lichfield 10k and Badgers Atherstone 10k.

WALES
▶ **Cardiff Bay 10k:** This is a favourite with our Welsh contingent because it is a 'lovely, flat route with beautiful views,' according to Hayley Norris.

Also highly rated is the Powys 10k trail in Welshpool.

SCOTLAND
▶ **Loch Ness 10k:** This race is favoured by many including Fee FG for its 'beautiful scenery and amazing atmosphere.'

▶ **City of Stirling 10k:** Sheila Taylor is among the fans of this race. She says: 'It's surrounded by absolutely beautiful scenery such as Stirling castle, the Wallace monument, the Ochil hills and the Forth river. There's also a great T-shirt and a caramel wafer at the end.'

▶ **Balmoral 10k:** The royals love Balmoral and so do our runners! Nicola Harrison says that the race has 'stunning views and an almighty hill in the middle', while Andrea Watt adds: 'The best 10k I've ever done! Beautiful course and views.'

Also highly rated are Glasgow Women's 10k and Great Scottish Run, both organised by the Great Run Company on routes in Glasgow.

NORTHERN IRELAND

▶ **Causeway Coast 10k:** This is a trail run along the coastal path on the north coast of Northern Ireland, parts of it on the Giant's Causeway World Heritage site. Fiona Ann Patterson says: 'The route is like no other. It is pretty much a single path over stiles, up and down steps, running along a beach and through dunes, but the views are amazing. I couldn't believe it when I reached the 5k mark as I was having such fun.'

Also highly recommended is Craic 10k held on St Patrick's Day in Belfast.

MULTIPLE LOCATIONS

▶ **Women's Running 10k:** These races are held throughout the UK, organised by the magazine of the same name. RMR members like Leanne Verduyn say they enjoy them because they have a 'great atmosphere, all-female participants and a nice goody bag and bling!'

▶**Jane Tomlinson's Run For All**: Races from 10k to Half Marathon organised around the UK including Leeds, Nottingham and York in memory of running enthusiast, Jane, who died of cancer in 2007. Michelle Ward says she loves the events as they have 'a fantastic atmosphere and some really inspirational people of all abilities that take part,' while Anne-Marie Readman says that they are 'all fun and accessible'.

▶**Great Run series**: Their most famous events are the longer-distance Great North Run (13.1 miles) and Great South Run (10 miles), but they also organise a number of 10ks around the country which come highly recommended by RMR members of all abilities for their organisation and atmosphere.

RMR MEMBERS REVEAL THEIR FAVOURITE UK HALF MARATHONS

We asked RMR members to reveal their favourite half marathons in the UK. Here are the ones that came out top, divided by region.

SOUTH OF ENGLAND
▶**Royal Parks Half**: Starting and finishing in leafy Hyde Park, London, when the autumn colours are in their prime, this race got a lot of votes because members loved the cheering crowds and beautiful scenery. Fiona Sawkill said 'it's just wonderful in so many ways', while Marie Boddington said 'I

will never forget the noise as you come back into the park at mile six. The support was amazing all the way round.'

▶ **Reading Half**: This springtime half marathon, which ends in the town's football club stadium, offers a varied course which attracts both first-timers and elite athletes. Naomi Creaser says that 'the finish in the stadium is fab', while Janice Phelan says 'the support from the locals throughout is unreal! And it's a good route.' Heather Talbot adds: 'Reading is my favourite by far – I love the support, the bands, the beer at mile eight and the stadium finish.'

▶ **Bath Half**: Another flat and well-supported half, this two-lap course is also given the thumbs up because it has lots of PB potential. It's usually held in March so is popular with those training for a spring marathon. Leanne Weston says: 'The Bath Half is amazing with all its bands and supporters.'

▶ **Cambridge Half:** This half grows in popularity year on year and is a firm favourite with RMR members. The course winds through the historic university city and around surrounding rural villages. Dawn Pammenter says it's her top choice because of the 'great crowds'.

▶ **Fleet Half**: This well-established spring half bills itself as a 'pre-London-Marathon' event, so it attracts many who are preparing to run 26.2 miles as well as those targeting the shorter distance. Helen Hart says she loves it because it's 'organised by runners for runners. Great course, fabulous local support and friendly marshals. And it's not too big — there are enough people to create a great atmosphere but it doesn't take half an hour to cross the start line.'

▶ **Hastings Half:** This is a popular place for runners to do battle with their PBs. Fans include Nadia Winborn who says: 'It's a little hilly but the support of the spectators is amazing.' Rachael Hogan agrees: 'Up that huge hill, then a lovely few miles down to the finish. Lovely locals with fresh oranges for the runners.'

NORTH OF ENGLAND

▶ **The Great North Run:** 'No contest,' declared Clur Geebrand when voting the Great North as her favourite half. The iconic race starts in Newcastle and finishes beside the sea in South Shields with enthusiastic crowds lining the entire course. Madeleine Vernon says: 'My favourite half has to be the Great North Run… the cheers, the crowds, the locals offering everything from jelly babies to digestives and beer at 11.5 miles!' Kerry Curtis agrees, saying: 'It was amazing — I loved the route and the support.' Amanda Copcutt Lunn adds: 'Love the Great North. Very crowded but a wonderful atmosphere!'

▶ **Liverpool Half:** Maureen Dunn is among those who love this mass-participation race held every May. Organised by runrocknroll.com, there's plenty of music to enjoy along the large loop of the city. Maureen says: 'It's a great course, well organised with a fantastic atmosphere.' Diane Sylvester agrees, saying the route is 'a good mix of city, parks, music, and of course running along the River Mersey to the finish line!'

▶ **Keswick Half:** This half in the Lake District is said to be one of the most scenic in the country, as the route passes picturesque Derwentwater and the Newlands Valley. Lisa Gilbert is among those who say the challenging course is not to be missed because it is 'hilly but beautiful'.

MIDLANDS
▶ **Lincoln Half:** This autumn half starts and finishes at the showground, and the course offers a tour of the beautiful city's sights, including the cathedral. Katie Griffiths says she recommends it because there's 'great crowd support and a slight challenge too with a hill on the route.'

▶ **Turkey Trot:** Held in the village of Keyworth in Nottinghamshire every December, this half always sells out fast despite the undulating course and likelihood of wintry weather. Beth Rushton says it always helps her feel festive, especially as turkeys are given out as prizes! She says of the race: 'It's freezing cold and has some hills, but it always produces PBs and, for me, it marks the start of Christmas.'

▶ **Ramathon Derby Half:** There's a lot of love for this June half marathon in Derby. Leyla Brooke says it's her favourite because the course has 'so much variety, from roads to canals!' She adds: 'I love it! It's so well organised with loads of support from the crowds.'

WALES

▶ **Cardiff Half**: With a fast course offering the chance to gain a PB, RMR members love the atmosphere at this event. Jodie Evans says it's an 'amazing one' because 'it is so inclusive for everyone, not just elites. The crowds stay out and everyone is so friendly.' Cat Lane said she agreed '100 per cent'. 'I'm hooked. This year it will be my fourth run there,' she added.

▶ **Conwy Half**: This is another Welsh half popular with RMR members. Alexandra Galloway says she recommends it for the 'superb scenery. There's a brutal hill but who wants this to be easy?'

SCOTLAND

▶ **Mamores Half**: This off-road half in the Scottish Highland village of Glen Coe has breath-taking scenery. Gillian Ross describes the run as 'amazingly beautiful'. Ruth Crawford agrees: 'Seconded, just amazing!'

▶ **Edinburgh Half**: Part of the city's Marathon Festival, this half gives people the chance to experience the atmosphere of the celebrated Edinburgh Marathon without having to run as far.

Laura Riddell says it is her favourite as she 'loves the fact it starts with a downhill' and has a 'great atmosphere'.

NORTHERN IRELAND

▶ **Causeway Coast Half**: This off-road half is part of a 26Extreme-organised event which also gives you the option of running a 10k (as recommended in the 10k section), a marathon or an ultra. It comes highly recommended for the stunning surroundings. Sharon Kennedy says: 'It's a testing half starting in *Game Of Thrones* territory ('the Iron Islands') along a heart-stopping cliff path through an area of outstanding natural beauty. There're breath-taking views of one of the wonders of the natural world – the limestone columns of World Heritage Site, The Giant's Causeway. I doubt there's another half anywhere that matches the spectacular scenery.'

▶ **Larne Half:** This March race is recommended for virgin half marathoners and more experienced runners alike. It runs along the coast road offering pretty sea views. Fiona McDonald says: 'It's good for a first half marathon as it's fairly flat. There's great scenery and the weather is likely to be nice and cool as it's in March.'

▶ **Ards Half:** Part of the Pure Running Half Marathon series in June, this undulating half is run on the North Down coast in the shadow of Scrabo Tower. Siobhan Grant says: 'What stands out about Ards Half is the level of support and encouragement around the course from the local club's marshals – they make this event what it is. On every corner over the full 13.1 miles, there was unending encouragement for everyone, even back to those like me who would finish in the last fifty. The tough climbs are soon forgotten once you finish as you experience the incredible post-race hospitality of hot food and doughnuts, to name but a few highlights.'

We asked RMR members to vote for their favourite race distance and here is the result...
1. 10k
2. Half Marathon
3. 5k
4. Marathon
5. Ultramarathon

TOP TIPS FOR RACE SUCCESS

Once you've signed up for a race you're bound to feel a mix of excitement, nerves and anticipation, which will only increase the closer you get to the big day. If you're a virgin racer, you might be wondering what to expect. Or, if you've raced before, perhaps you want some hints on how to improve. Here is our advice on how to enhance your race-day experience.

IN THE BUILD-UP
First of all you have to decide which race you want to target – a long or short distance, a mass road run, a smaller local fun run or an off-road trail race? The choice is yours! Just consider how much time you have to train and what you think you're capable of in the time you have available. Also, think about what you might enjoy more: running somewhere with spectacular scenery, having lots of crowds to cheer you on or being part of a small event where it won't be as busy.

If you are targeting a shorter distance, such as 5k–10k, allow six to nine weeks to train for it. For a longer-distance run, like a half, a marathon or an ultra, you'll need to start training 12–15 weeks ahead of race day. You will probably find it easier to train if you follow a schedule. We have some at the back of this book (page 262), while many are also available online. You could also consider hiring a running coach who could do a bespoke plan for you.

If you want to run well you will have to be dedicated to training, but don't worry if you have to miss the odd session due to illness or life getting in the way. Just try to do your best with the time you have.

Do some training runs in the kit you intend to race in to ensure it's comfortable. You could put your name or nickname on your vest as many find this helps give them a boost as spectators can pick them out to cheer them on personally. Numerous companies offer this service, or you can stitch or write it on yourself in marker pen.

THE WEEK BEFORE

The butterflies in your stomach will start fluttering this week and intensify on race day, but don't worry – it's completely normal. Your body is producing adrenaline and this will actually help you run as it can increase blood-flow to the muscles. It's known as the fight-or-flight response, which helped early humans to survive by giving them the ability to either fight danger or to run from it, so the surge of adrenaline you feel is an evolutionary aid to help your body perform at its highest level.

Don't train too hard in the final week as you want to be fresh and full of energy for race day. If you've missed any training, then by this point it's too late to make up for it and you'd be better off conserving your energy in order to race well rather than trying to cram in extra sessions. Reducing your training as race-day gets closer is known as tapering, and the length of your taper will vary depending on the race distance you're preparing for. Marathoners should have a three-week taper (see more on this in the marathon section later in the chapter), but when racing a shorter distance, just easing down a few days before the event is adequate.

Make sure you get plenty of sleep this week. The night before you might find you don't sleep well due to nerves and worries about the race or missing the start. You might also have to get up extra early to eat breakfast and to get to the event in plenty of time. As long as you can get some high-quality sleep in the week of the race, you shouldn't be hindered if your sleep the night before the big day isn't as good as it could be.

THE NIGHT BEFORE

Have a good meal containing some carbs the evening before the race (see chapter six, page 211, for more on this). Stick to drinking water and avoid alcohol as it can dehydrate you – save the champagne for the post-race celebration!

Prepare your kit and pack your bag so you're ready to go and not rushing around getting stressed in the morning. You might worry about getting up on time or oversleeping (although perhaps not if you have young children!), so if necessary set more than one alarm. If you are staying in a hotel, arrange a wake-up call.

Plan how you will get to the event and allow extra time to deal with unforeseen circumstances, such as a train being cancelled or getting stuck in traffic.

If you have been sent a map of the course then familiarise yourself with it. Knowing the route might help you break up the race mentally, and you can work out where the drink stations and toilets are along the way, should you need them. Finding out the course elevation will also prepare you for any up-hill climbs that might be on the route. If your family are going with you, find out where they will stand on the course to watch you so you can look out for them. Knowing where they will be can incentivise you to get to that point.

Make sure you also discuss where you will meet them afterwards. If you're not carrying your mobile while you run, you'll have no means of contacting them when you finish, and even if you do have your phone, at some large events the networks get so busy in the area, you won't get through anyway. If it's a big race it's inadvisable to arrange to meet 'at the finish' because there are so many people you'll never find each other. Some races have designated meet-up areas, but if yours doesn't, pick your own spot by finding a distinctive landmark.

RACE-DAY CHECKLIST

The night before the race, make sure you have packed (or have put out, ready to wear) the following:

▶ **Running shorts/leggings and vest with race number** (and your ICE details) pinned on
▶ **Trainers**
▶ **Chiptiming device** (if provided) ready to be attached to the laces of your trainers or wrapped round your ankle. Some events incorporate the chip into the race number
▶ **Running socks**, plus a spare pair so you can put dry ones on after the race
▶ **Charged up device**, if using e.g. stopwatch, GPS, heart rate monitor
▶ **Clothes to keep you warm** before and after the race e.g. T-shirt, jumper, jogging bottoms, waterproof jacket etc.
▶ **Kit bag** – some races will provide these; if so make sure your number is displayed on it
▶ **Spare safety pins/bib clips** in case you lose one or forget to pin your number onto your vest!
▶ **Disposable clothes/bin bag** to wear in case you have to hand in your kit bag early but want to keep warm before the start

▶ **Water** to keep sipping before and after the race. You can then leave this with your kit when running and use water stations on the course to stay hydrated. If you prefer to race while carrying your own water, make sure you pack a bottle you find it easy to run with

▶ **Weather dependent accessories** – if it's going to be cold, hat and gloves. If hot, sun cream, cap and sweatbands

▶ **Snacks** for after the race, preferably high in protein to aid recovery e.g. nuts, or a treat to motivate you to reach the finish!

▶ **Toilet roll and/or wet wipes**, as they often run out in the facilities at the start. Wet wipes will help you freshen up after the race if you get very sweaty

▶ **Gels** – both anti-chafing so you can touch up any bits that might rub when you get to the course, and energy gels if you intend to take these when racing

▶ **Change of underwear** for after the race as what you run in will get sweaty

▶ **Fully charged mobile phone** so you can take selfies before and after to share with RMR!

THE MORNING OF THE RACE

Ensure you have everything on our checklist. Get up with enough time to eat breakfast – such as porridge or toast – at least two hours before the race start so it's fully digested by the time you run. Drink water, and you could also have a tea or coffee — caffeine has been proven to boost performance (but make sure not to overdo it as tea and coffee are also diuretics).

When you get dressed, smother anti-chafing gel anywhere you think your shoes or clothing might rub.

Get to the course at least an hour before the start so you have time to go to the toilet (expect long queues!), leave your kit bag (races usually provide secure areas for this, or trucks to take bags to the finish if it's in a different place to the start) and warm up (a short, gentle jog) without feeling stressed.

Don't get too cold before the race starts by keeping extra layers on for as long as possible. If you do have to hand your kit bag in and head to the line early, wear an old T-shirt or bin bag to keep you warm in the meantime (these will also keep you drier if it's raining). Strip it off at the last minute but dispose of this garment or bag responsibly — both to avoid littering and to prevent someone running behind you tripping over your discarded item. You could hand it to someone who you know nearby, or throw it in a bin. Some races collect old T-shirts left at the start to give to charity, so check if this is an option too.

SHOWTIME!

Once you are instructed to head to the start line, check to see if it has been marked out with positions for predicted finish times. If you were asked to give your expected time when you entered the race you may have already been given a zone to start in. If you're not expecting to be one of the fastest participants, don't be tempted to move forward so you are closer to the line. As long as the race is chip timed you will get an accurate time regardless of how far you are from the line when the starting gun goes, as your chip won't be activated until you cross it. For this reason, your chip time is the most accurate and what counts as your PB rather than the 'gun time' (your finishing time from when the gun sounds to when you finish). In mass-participation races, gun times and chip times can be vastly different as it can take some runners a long time to reach the start line due to the sheer numbers up ahead. For example, at the Great North Run, the elite men have often finished before all of the slower runners have even made it over the start line!

It's best to start the race in the area suitable for your pace so you don't impede faster runners who might be behind you, and so you can fall into a rhythm with those around you who will be of a similar ability. If you start too far forward, you might find it demoralising if those who were standing beside you at the start speed away, or if you keep getting overtaken by faster runners coming up behind you.

DURING THE RACE

Here are some top tips for running at your best and having an enjoyable experience once the race gets under way.

▶ **Pace yourself:** It is imperative when racing not to start off too fast! If you do, you risk overexerting yourself and struggling to finish. Failing to pace yourself and paying for it later is expressed in various terms, such as 'blowing up' or 'bonking' and, in the case of marathon running, can contribute to you 'hitting the wall'. Try to work out in advance what your race pace is based on your training runs and your target finishing time. For example, if you want to finish a 10k in under 50 minutes, you need to run at a pace of five minutes per kilometre, (or eight minutes per mile). If you want to break an hour, then aim for a six-minute-per-kilometre (or 9.30-minute-per-mile) pace. If you have a GPS watch, you can check your own pace as you run, or if you use a stopwatch and the course has mile-markers, you can check the elapsed time for each mile. If not, some events hire pacemakers to take part. They'll usually run carrying giant signs advertising the pace they're running at, so you can look out for one you can follow. Alternatively, just judge your pace from how your body feels with your brain in check – it will feel easy at the start because your legs are fresh and raring to go and the adrenaline will be pumping through your body. So just make sure you are running at a pace that's both comfortable and one that you can sustain for the entire race distance. If you've gone off slow and feel like you have more to give you can pick up the pace in the second half of the race. You will feel better if you can run a 'negative split' in this way, which means running the second half of the race faster than the first half. It's called negative, but it can make for a much more positive experience, as RMR member Lucy Bailie discovered. She said: 'During the London Marathon I told myself "in the first half don't be an idiot, in the second half don't be a wimp." It helped me slow my pace in the first few miles and kept me going in the last five. My stats showed that I passed over one thousand people in my last seven kilometres and only thirty-four passed me, which suggests they didn't take the advice and went off too fast!'

▶ **Think positive:** Getting through a race can often be down to your mental strength as well as your physical endurance. Having a positive mindset will help you keep going. Try repeating a mantra in your head and remember why you are running. Perhaps you are raising money for charity or to prove you can achieve a target you've set yourself. Whatever your reason, let it motivate you to keep going. You could also try strategies like breaking the race up into chunks to make achieving the total distance more manageable. This worked for Katherine Ireson. She said: 'The best tip I have heard is "run the mile you're in." It means you don't think too much about the whole thing. That certainly helped me during the London Marathon.'

▶ **Stay hydrated and topped-up with fuel:** If you're doing a short race and it isn't a hot day then drinking before and after the run will be adequate. However, if it's hot and you're running far, you'll need to drink during the race as well, and might need to take energy gels and drinks to keep you going. See more on this in chapter six.

▶ **Enjoy it!** We can often get so hung-up on achieving times and distances we forget to simply appreciate the joy of running surrounded by others. Allow yourself to soak up the race atmosphere, smile and be proud of what you are doing.

AFTER THE RACE

Get some warm clothes on and change out of anything that's damp. If you haven't raced in compression garments, putting them on now could aid your recovery. Make sure you keep drinking to replenish any fluids lost and try to eat within an hour of finishing. Go for something high in protein which will help with muscle repair (see chapter six, page 205).

If the race hasn't gone as well as you'd hoped then try not to be disheartened. Think about what went wrong and how you can improve next time, and remember that racing well can be down to trial and error. There are plenty more races out there, so if you missed out on a PB or feel you didn't do yourself justice, try again next time.

Whatever happens, whether you ran a PB or not, celebrate your achievement. Finishing any race isn't easy and you deserve to give yourself a pat on the back for all the training you've done and for having the guts and determination to take part. Get your finishing medal and show it off with pride!

More race tips from RMR members…

'Run your own race.'
Beverley Packwood

'When I'm struggling, I start to repeat the mantra: "I am strong, I am invincible". I find it really helps distract me from negative thoughts and stops me from slowing down.'
Naomi Creaser

'I always say in my head: "You're strong, you love hills!" Plus I try to never stop and walk in a race because mentally that finishes me off.'
Nicola Carter

'My mantra is and always will be: "She believed she could and she did." I think running is fifty per cent physical fifty per cent mental – once you believe you can, you will!'
Claire Daniels

'I've found when I am struggling mentally during a race, concentrating on my cadence keeps me going on pace... 1-2-1-2-1-2-1-2 etc. Also: smile, high-five kids and enjoy picking people off near the end of the race.'
Jenevieve Newman Beavers

'For a fabulous race, it's all about mind and attitude, I've discovered. If you think you can, you can. Simple as. If you think you can't, you'll probably struggle. It sounds easy but it's hard to do. However, if you are working on your running form, speed and distance, why can't you be working equally hard on your mindset?'
Kate Losowsky

'When someone says you can't, turn around and say: "Watch me!"'
Tracey Francis

GOING THE DISTANCE: ADVICE ON RUNNING A MARATHON

When tackling a marathon many of the race-day tips outlined previously apply, but there are also some additional considerations. A marathon is such a long way that you need to be fully prepared by doing the correct training and by following a sensible strategy on race day.

TRAINING FOR A MARATHON

When it comes to training, you'll need at least 12–15 weeks to prepare, depending on your current level of fitness. You shouldn't just go out and do a long run – you need to build up to it. Where you start will depend on your current level of fitness and how far you have run before. Whatever your ability, you should work towards doing 20 miles in training. In the first few weeks of your plan you might start by doing ten miles and then do an extra mile each week. Increasing your long run gradually in this way will help you to get used to running further and decrease your chances of getting injured. The first time you do a run that's longer than one you've ever done before, such as 16 miles, you might struggle and wonder how you'll be able to manage another ten. At these times, trust in your training. It's amazing how the body can adapt, and each week you'll find you are increasing in stamina. Don't forget that on race day you'll also have adrenaline, cheering crowds and other runners pulling you along which will make a big difference.

The long run is crucial in marathon training so you'll have to be committed to fitting one in every week. It can be difficult to run for a long time alone, so join a group run if you can. If you don't have anyone to train with, in the build-up to spring and autumn marathons there are some 20-mile training runs and races organised around the country that you could join in with. You could also try to convince your partner to come with you on a bike. If you have a friend who is a runner but not training for a marathon they could join you for an hour so you're not doing the whole thing solo, and this would also help you break up the distance.

Most training plans will cap the long run at 20 miles. You might think this is illogical when the race is another 10k, but experts believe that going further in training is counter-productive. Trying to run the full marathon distance, or close to it, could make you too exhausted and cause too much muscle damage ahead of the big day. However, training up to 20 miles will get your body used to running a long way and give you 'time on your feet' to make your legs stronger. By tapering (more on this in the next section), pacing yourself and taking on adequate water and fuel on race day (see chapter six including the section on carb-loading on page 211), you'll be able to manage the last six miles.

During your marathon training, you might find you have to make other sacrifices in order to succeed. You might have to miss a certain night out to do your long run the next day without a hangover, or cut back on eating certain unhealthy foods such as greasy takeaways that could upset your stomach when running. You will have to be dedicated to your training, but remember it is only for a few months and it will be worth it when you have that shiny medal around your neck.

Enter one or two shorter races such as a half marathon in the build-up to the marathon so you can practise your race-day routine. This is the time to see if your kit is comfortable and to work out which energy gels or drinks you prefer. Try to fit this race in about halfway into your training schedule so you will be recovered from it by marathon day. It will also give you a much-needed boost to keep you motivated; once you've experienced the race atmosphere, you'll be keen to do it all again and it could give you a new sense of vigour towards your remaining marathon training. It will also help you learn what pace you might be capable of running the marathon in.

TAPERING

With three weeks to go until the marathon, you should start to 'taper' which means easing back on your training. Each week your mileage should be less so that your legs are fresh and you have plenty of energy by the big day. So, for example, your long run a fortnight before the marathon could be reduced to around 15 miles, and with a week to go, to eight or nine miles. You should also decrease the length and intensity of your other runs.

In the final week before the race you shouldn't be doing too much training at all. Take extra rest days if you need them and just do some short, easy runs to keep your legs ticking over on the days you do train. You might start to feel a little sluggish and even lazy after all the hard training you have been doing, but it is important to be well-rested so you're in prime shape for taking on the marathon. Don't worry about losing any fitness – you won't in such a short space of time. Instead, revel in having the perfect excuse to avoid doing any housework for a week!

You might also start experiencing what runners jokingly refer to as 'maranoia' during this time. You might suddenly start to feel ill or to worry that a niggle in your muscle is going to stop you being able to run. Often this is just your mind playing tricks on you as you obsess about what lies ahead. If you are concerned, though, visit your GP or a physio. If they find you do have an issue that will curtail your race plans, then consider pulling out. It can be difficult to make this decision but you have to put your health first. If you are too ill or injured to race, then you might be able to defer your place and run next year. Remember, there will be other races, and it is far better to run when you can be at your best than to limp round and have a terrible experience.

RACE DAY

If you do make it to the start line, full of nerves and as ready as you'll ever be (see the tips on how to prepare the night before the race and the kit checklist on pages 167–170) the most important thing to keep in mind when it comes to the marathon is not to go off too fast. If you begin too quickly in a 5k or 10k you might get away with it, or only find you struggle for a short time. However, if you do it in a marathon, you can feel awful and suffer from cramp and fatigue when you still have many more miles to go. This is why the term 'hitting the wall' is often associated with marathoners. Many who experience it have gone off too fast and run out of energy, especially if they haven't taken on enough fuel to keep them going. 'Hitting the wall' can ruin your marathon experience and might even prevent you finishing. Try to avoid it by preparing for the run with adequate training, by pacing yourself and by eating and drinking enough before and during the race.

Many say that, when it comes to the marathon, the race actually begins at 20 miles, because if you've made it that far you have to dig deep to keep going. At this point it will become a mental struggle as well as a physical one, so RMR's Bernie Bird shares how she coped: 'Instead of dreading the last six miles and expecting it to be hard, I just visualised my usual 10k run (around the big block) and kept saying to myself: "It's just around the block." When I got to the last three miles, I changed it to "round the little block". It worked! Many also like to think at 5k that there's "only a parkrun to go".'

Taking part in the marathon can be a truly unforgettable and emotional experience and you'll have ups and downs in this race unlike you'll have in any other. At times you might think you'll never make it to the end and wonder why you signed up to do it in the first place. Remember to keep believing in yourself. Break the race up if you have to so it doesn't seem as daunting. Just focus on getting to five miles, then ten miles rather than thinking about reaching 26.2. If you do find it's too much and you have to stop and walk then don't be afraid to do so. As explained in chapter two on 'Jeffing' (page 53), some find run-walking leads to a better time than trying to run the whole way.

Many RMR members compare running a marathon to childbirth! It hurts like hell but it is worth it, and when you cross the finish line you'll experience an overwhelming sense of pride and achievement. RMR's Nicola Carter knows this feeling well. She says: 'Finishing a race is the best feeling ever. I feel very lucky to be able to run at all after a health scare four years ago. Every race, no matter what the time, is a personal triumph. It makes me feel alive.'

RECOVERING FROM A MARATHON

Often you soon forget about the pain of finishing a marathon and think: 'When can I do this again?' If you are keen to do another marathon, make sure you give yourself adequate time to recover first. There are some amazing individuals who have pulled off some admirable feats of endurance by doing multiple marathons back-to-back, but it is usually advisable to stick to doing only one or two a year to avoid putting too much stress and strain on your body.

Allowing yourself time to recover is particularly important after a marathon as during the long-distance run you can cause micro-tears to your muscles. You might also have rubbed blisters, chafed areas of skin or mentally exhausted yourself. Take time to celebrate your achievement and have a few days off from doing any exercise. After that, you could try doing some 'active recovery', such as swimming and walking, which will help to alleviate muscle pain without causing too much stress. It's also perfectly normal and expected to feel stiff and sore after the marathon. You might struggle to walk up and down the stairs and even something as simple as pulling your socks on will feel like an immense effort. It's all part of the recovery process, so be kind to your body at this time. Try soaking in a hot bath, wearing compression clothing or getting a gentle massage.

When you do resume running, take it easy at first – you might find your legs are still a little sore. They could still feel heavy weeks later, so be patient – you have run a marathon! It is a fantastic feat to achieve. Once you've completed 26.2 miles you're forever in the club of being a 'marathoner' and that's something to be very proud of indeed.

RMR MEMBERS REVEAL THEIR FAVOURITE MARATHONS

When we asked members to put forward their favourite marathon, perhaps unsurprisingly, the London Marathon received the most votes. It's a true celebration of running, from the world's best long-distance athletes at the front, to the charity runners weighed down by eccentric fancy dress at the back, and all the club runners and fundraisers giving their all in between. The course takes in many famous London landmarks, including crossing over Tower Bridge, passing the Tower of London and Big Ben, and finishing in front of Buckingham Palace. As the coverage of the race is so widespread, you'll really feel like you are part of something big, and you'll probably find that non-running friends, family and colleagues will follow it too, even though they might be oblivious to other races at other times of the year. Theresa Waller says she loves the London Marathon because of the 'amazing support and iconic views', while Rebecca Howells said: 'It was totally awesome. I felt euphoric during and afterwards, and I was still smiling weeks later.'

Other UK road marathons popular with RMR members are Manchester, Brighton, Edinburgh and Chester. A large contingent also recommend Milton Keynes. One of them is Jo Robinson, who says it has 'a nice mix of road and park paths and a great medal. The start is in waves so the course isn't too crowded, and there's a great finish in the stadium.' Meanwhile, for a scenic road marathon, Loch Ness comes highly rated.

Recommended trail marathons include Beachy Head in Eastbourne, The Moyleman in Lewes, The Longhorn, Nottinghamshire, and Kielder and Windermere Marathons, both in the Lake District. RMR's Tinu Ogundari likes the latter so much, she's done it 14 times! 'The scenery is to die for – it's just the perfect location to hold such an event,' she said.

For those willing to travel abroad for a marathon, RMR members recommend ones held in Paris, New York, Dublin and Walt Disney World, Florida.

GETTING A PLACE IN THE LONDON MARATHON

The London Marathon isn't just popular with RMR members, it's also one of the world's most famous races. Getting one of the 40,000 places is so coveted, a ballot is in place to try to ensure a fair distribution. In 2017, a world-record number of 386,050 applicants entered the ballot from the UK and overseas. The ballot usually opens in May and applicants find out in October if they have successfully gained a spot. RMR members often speculate as to whether there's a way to increase your chances by putting down a certain predicted finishing time, but it's all down to the luck of the draw. If you aren't lucky enough to get a place then don't despair as there are other ways you could still take part.

▶**Run for charity:** The London Marathon is the country's largest fundraising event and every year places are reserved for charities. If you are willing to raise money via sponsorship then you could apply for one of these spots. Contact individual charities to find out how to apply for their places. Many will ask you to raise a minimum amount of money in return for the place, such as £1,000–£2,000. It can be a big commitment to raise this kind of money, so consider if you can take the time and effort to do this alongside your training. Read fundraising tips from RMR members in chapter seven, page 236.

▶**Gain a club place:** Running clubs associated with British Athletics can be given up to four places each year (the number of places allocated depends on the size of the club's membership). It's down to each club to decide how they distribute these places. This is another good reason to join a running club, as you've got to be in it to win it!

▶**Achieve a fast time:** The London Marathon (and some other big-city marathons) reserve places every year for those who have a 'good for age' or 'championship' time. You could achieve this time at a different marathon as long as it meets their entry standards. Check the London Marathon website for up-to-date information on their qualifying times and how to enter. At the time of writing, the Good For Age and Championship requirements for women are as follows…

AGE	QUALIFYING TIME
18–40	Sub 3:45
41–49	Sub 3:50
50–59	Sub 4:00
60–64	Sub 4:30
65–69	Sub 5:00
70–75	Sub 6:00
76+	Sub 6:30
CHAMPIONSHIP	Sub 3:15 (or a recent half in sub 90 minutes)
ELITE	By invitation only; for those who have proven they are capable of a super-fast time, usually sub 2 hours 40 minutes. The elite women start earlier than the mass field and are often competing for places in championships like the Olympics.

Note that the times above are to the second. If, for example, you have run a time of 3:45.01, you won't be eligible for a GFA place.

Remember, if you don't get a place in London then there are plenty of other marathons with a similar atmosphere where you could have an equally enjoyable experience. Check out the other marathons recommended by RMR members earlier in the chapter (page 184). By entering a different one you might even achieve a Good For Age or Championship time so you can apply for London the next time around. You might even find you enjoy the other event so much that you're not so bothered about doing London anymore and would rather do the other marathon again. If you do want to experience running through the capital then there are also other races staged on central London roads throughout the year you could do instead, such as the London Winter Run and Royal Parks Half.

ULTRA RUNNING

Ultra running – which means racing a distance beyond 26.2 miles – has really taken off in recent years. There's no limit to how far an ultra run can be: some are 50 miles, some are 100 miles and some are several hundreds of miles long. In some, participants will be expected to run continuously, which means running through the night without sleeping, whereas others are 'multi-stage events' broken up with camping overnight. Some involve running a set distance, while others involve running as far as you can within a given time, such as 12 hours.

When preparing for an ultra event, many of the rules of marathon training and racing still apply, but you might need to give yourself a few weeks' extra training to prepare. The long run is, again, crucial but just like you don't need to run 26.2 miles ahead of a marathon, you don't need to do the full distance of your ultra in one go. Just do plenty of long-distance runs to give yourself 'time on your feet'. You might also want to do some long-distance training walks, or a combination of long run-walks, since it's likely that you'll need to spend some sections of the race walking.

Taking on food and drink as you go is essential in order to keep going. Most ultra races will have stations where they provide food and drink. However, it's advisable to also carry your own in case you feel weak in between stations. To avoid a stitch, stomach upset or indigestion, experiment with what you eat and drink in training to find the best products and foods for you. To make carrying enough fluid easier, you can get hydration packs which enable you to carry the water on your back and sip it through an attached straw. If you decide to do this, practise running with it on in training (the same goes for any backpack or bum bag you might race in) so you can get used to moving with the weight.

Wearing comfortable kit and liberally applying anti-chafing gel is a must, but it's likely you will still get some blisters or rubbed skin due to the length of time you'll be running. You might also find it best to wear trainers in a larger size than normal as your feet can swell during an ultra, and making this adjustment could minimise rubbing from too-tight shoes.

Remember: an ultra isn't something to sign up for without serious consideration first, and if you do want to do one you need to be fully committed to train for it. As well as covering long distances, some will also be over difficult terrain.

Some are so tricky that you're allowed to be supported by a 'crew'. This small group might be allowed to run with you on certain sections and can give you extra food and drink and a change of kit – since there will be only so much you can carry yourself – and generally give you the support and encouragement you need to keep going. Choose your crew wisely; they will need to have enough stamina to be there for you as long as your run takes and the patience to put up with you if you start to get grumpy as you fatigue!

Doing an ultra can be a great adventure but can also put a large strain on your body, so always ensure you are properly prepared and in the best of health and fitness to do one.

OBSTACLE COURSE RACES

If you want to try something a bit different then an obstacle course race could be for you! They can involve anything from clambering over giant walls or crawling under nets to swinging across monkey bars. The races can be hard work but a lot of fun. You often also run as a team, and helping one another along the way creates great camaraderie between you all. Events can vary in distance but it's not all about achieving a good time – the accomplishment is completing the obstacle course. They can vary in difficulty, so do some research first to ensure they are suitable for your level of fitness if you are worried. Cancer Research UK's Pretty Muddy is a gentle introduction to obstacle races and is suitable for all abilities.

CROSS COUNTRY AND TRAIL RUNNING

Cross country and trail racing are other ways to have an interesting change from the roads. Although they both mean running off road, there are subtle differences between the two. Cross country racing usually involves competing in historic leagues around the country, and entry is often only open to members of running clubs who are in that league. The season runs from October to March and one of the main events is the National Cross Country Championship in February, when all the clubs from around the country come together to compete for individual and team honours. Hundreds take part and seeing them all stampede at the start is quite a spectacle! The races tend to be 6–8 kilometres long for women. Some leagues will run the men and women together, others will have separate races. There are often separate junior races for under 11s–under 20s too, so it's a good way to get your children involved.

Courses are run in parks, fields and forests and often involve hills and lots of mud! You might have to jump across a ditch, run through a brook or steeplechase a fallen log along the way. As the races are held in autumn and winter the weather is often cold and wet too, but races are very rarely cancelled, even if it snows, as cross country spikes and trail shoes give extra grip if the ground is slippery. PBs and times aren't important in cross country racing and it's even difficult to compare course records, as conditions under-foot on the same route can be very changeable depending on the weather.

Once again, competing in a cross country race is open to all abilities so don't let being a slower runner put you off. It can be great fun to splash through the mud and you can run without the worry of pace and mile splits, as courses don't have mile or kilometre markers like most road races. A cross country race is an opportunity to embrace the childlike joy of running outdoors, and if you want to be competitive you can see how many others you can beat. The hills and uneven terrain are also great for improving stamina and leg strength.

The same goes for trail running, a term that encompasses any running and racing done off road. Trail races can be any length and staged at any time of year and, like with cross country running, your finishing time is less important – you are bound to be slower on trails than when covering the same distance on the road due to any steep uphill sections and rocky, muddy paths. Some trail races also won't have mile markers and might not even be marshalled, so you might have to navigate your own way. They will often involve spectacular scenery and wonderful views in rural locations, so trail racing is not to be missed if you'd like to experience an uplifting, exhilarating run.

VIRTUAL RACES

Unlike a traditional race, a virtual race doesn't involve joining in an event alongside others on a set date. Instead, participants are given a certain length of time to complete a distance, such as 5k. It means running your own personal 'race' on a route of your choosing, so it's perfect if you're looking for a gentle introduction to covering a certain distance or meeting a challenge. Lots of RMR members are big fans of virtual racing as it keeps them motivated, and can be more affordable and less intimidating than participating in a major event.

Once you have signed up for one (companies running virtual events include Virtual Runner UK and POW! Virtual Running), you decide when and where you'll do it. Afterwards, you send proof of your achievement, for example, by uploading a picture of the run as shown on your GPS watch, or on the monitor of a treadmill. The results can be shared with other entrants, so you can compete with others taking part.

Some virtual races can be run in one go and others require you to clock up the miles over a certain number of weeks. Some also ask participants to do the whole distance running, while others allow you to reach the target by walking, cycling or swimming too.

The funky medals you can win if you achieve the virtual race target are another plus-point.

BANISHING THE POST-RACE BLUES

After completing a race you have given up so much time to train for, it's not uncommon to feel a bit flat afterwards – both physically and mentally – after the initial high of finishing has worn off. Here are our tips on beating the post-race blues.

▶**Prepare to be pampered:** A race in which you have given your all can leave you feeling exhausted. If it was a long-distance event, your body will feel tired and achy and will need time to recover. Plan something in the week after the race to help rehabilitate you and to give you something relaxing to look forward to. You could plan a trip to a spa, a relaxing beach holiday or a weekend away.

▶**Beat the boredom:** If you were training for a long-distance event that required running lots of long, slow miles, you might feel a little bored of running. Stay interested in the sport by doing something completely different. Enter a short race which requires some speed work to train for it, or try an obstacle race where you might need to do some strength training in preparation. You could also try running on a completely different surface by entering a cross-country race or trail event. There's so much variety with running that, if you have become fed-up with one aspect, it's easy to find another way to make it still excite, interest and motivate you.

▶**Don't be down if you're still heavy-legged weeks later:** This feeling is completely normal, particularly if you have run a long race. You might find you still feel a bit sluggish weeks later and wonder if you will ever feel bouncy when running again. You will. Just be patient and allow your body to heal and get strong again by not trying to do too much too soon after a major race.

▶ **Keep your toe in the water:** If you've just completed a big challenge then you might physically need to take some time off from running to recover. But that doesn't mean stepping away completely from the sport you've grown to love. Why not volunteer at a race or parkrun, or help others get into running (see more on this in chapter seven, page 231).

▶ **Pick a new target:** If you find you've lost your running mojo post-race because having the event on the horizon was what was motivating you to train, then pick a new challenge to give you another goal to work towards. If you've just done a 5k, why not aim for another and try to go faster? Or try going longer by targeting a 10k or half marathon. You could also do a virtual race so you're still working towards something but can be more flexible about how you fit it into your life. Just make sure that, whatever you choose, it isn't too close to your last race (particularly if it was a long-distance event) so you have time to recover and then train again.

RMR STORIES

'For me, racing is about completing, not competing': RMR member Isobel Monaghan, 37, from Kingswinford, West Midlands, reveals how she overcame physical problems and her own mental barriers to become a marathoner.

As I crossed the finish line of the London Marathon, a friend made via RMR by my side, I couldn't believe what we had just achieved. It had been the most exciting, surreal, overwhelming and just altogether amazing experience of my life.

As a medal was hung round my neck, I couldn't believe that I could now say I was a marathoner. It felt incredible, not only because I had never considered myself to be athletic, but because just a few years before, I had been struggling to even walk.

Following the birth of my first son, Edward, in 2011, I was diagnosed with cauda equina syndrome (CES), a catastrophic herniated disc where the disc fragments compress the spinal cord. It seems it was brought on by the repetitive movement of bending and twisting to lift Edward from his cot, changing nappies on the floor and carrying the car-seat – all normal new mum tasks. I was just incredibly unlucky that a niggly bad back resulted in a prolapsed disc, and that the disc went into the spinal cord as opposed to in any other direction. As a result, I started suffering from terrible back pain with pins and needles and spasms like electric shocks. It was so bad that one day my husband, Lee, rushed me to A&E. I was advised to have surgery to relieve the pressure and prevent the symptoms worsening but I was warned I could be left unable to walk, and possibly unable to urinate without a catheter. It was a horrific diagnosis, but luckily my consultant was happy with the results of the surgery. However, I had lost the feeling in my left side. When I asked when it would return, I was told it may never do so. I was distraught.

After a week in hospital, I was discharged with a walking stick and moved with a strange, slow shuffle as I couldn't feel the ground with my left foot. Physiotherapy for three months helped improve my mobility but I had to learn to adapt my lifestyle. I needed to lean on a stick if I had to stand for longer than ten minutes. I could no longer drive a manual car, as my weakened left foot couldn't push the clutch pedal, and I had to clock-watch to make sure I went to the toilet regularly, as my brain couldn't receive signals telling me when I needed it. Despite how difficult my life now seemed, when I visited the consultant for a follow-up he was shocked I had even walked into the room unaided. He reassured me I was making excellent progress on the road to recovery, but neither of us would have believed that that path would take me to the start of the London Marathon!

Against all advice, and entirely unplanned, I then fell pregnant with twins. My weak body somehow managed to carry them to 37 weeks at which point I had a planned c-section, as there was no way my spine could risk the strain of labour. Everything was adjusted to help me cope with my beautiful newborns, Lucy and Arthur. I had car seats on wheels, the lightest pushchair I could buy and a raised playpen so I didn't have to bend.

My husband and family were a great help and my back gradually got stronger.

I decided I had to get fitter when the twins were three, and Edward four. My back problems had left me low in confidence and overweight. As my children were now all out of pushchairs and keen to explore the world, I knew I had to be fitter so I could keep up with them and keep them safe. I have never been sporty and I didn't even know if I would be able to run but I wanted to try, so I signed up for a Couch To 5k programme that was being run locally. The first week I couldn't even jog slowly for a minute. I had zero fitness and got hot and sweaty, huffing and puffing my way through each session despite it being a very cold January. But I kept going, and by April I was delighted to run my first 5k. Along with other women I met on the course, we decided to keep it up by doing our local parkrun regularly. It was then that someone added me to the Facebook group, Run Mummy Run. Everyone's enthusiasm for running was infectious and the support was incredible. No way was I going to stop running now.

The idea of racing made me feel sick with nerves but I plucked up the courage to do it to give myself goals to work towards. I read somewhere that it's about 'completing not competing' and I adopted that as my running motto. I ran a 10k and a half marathon and then entered the London Marathon ballot for 2017, caught up in the excitement of everyone else in RMR doing so. I was stunned months later when I discovered I had been given a place. At first I didn't want to tell anyone. It seemed ridiculous that I might run a marathon. I thought people would be upset with me, as I'd entered on a whim when serious runners – who had many more miles experience – had been unlucky time and time again. As it happens, my friends were all thrilled for me, and I vowed to take it seriously.

I followed a training plan as best as I could – having to skip runs sometimes due to the children getting ill, and the various other things that life throws at us. In the build-up I raced a half and a 20 miler, and I gradually increased my solo runs to ensure I was prepared.

The big day arrived and I met a group of RMR ladies at the start, pairing up with one of them – Caroline Robertson – who was a similar pace to me. From dashing for a last minute wee before the gun, to crossing the finish line in 5 hours 34 minutes, we ran every single step together. This is exactly what RMR is about for me: we supported one another all the way. I got two tiny blisters and a bit of muscle soreness but that was it. I didn't 'hit the wall' or experience any back pain. I was so proud of myself for finishing. Two days later life went on and I was back doing the school run and the ironing, but I was not the same. I was a marathoner!

Now I intend to carry on running and do lots more races. I still have a 'bad back' and I often get numbness down my left side, with my weak left foot affecting my gait. I am not built like a runner or elegant in any way, but that won't stop me because I love it. The distance is the achievement, not the time. I hope I can inspire others who are fearful of racing because they worry they are 'too slow'. The back of the pack has a lot of camaraderie, support and encouragement and so it's not a bad place to be! If you are nervous, start by joining in a mass-participation race such as the Great Run series as there you will see every age, ability, shape and size of runner. They are all-inclusive and I have never felt that I shouldn't be there. Although the start is daunting and you'll probably feel sick with nerves, trust me – the pride and sense of achievement at the end makes it all worthwhile.

CHAPTER SIX:
EAT, DRINK AND RUN MERRY

A HEALTHY BALANCE:
THE RECOMMENDED DAILY DIET

At RMR we don't believe in telling our members to go on starvation diets or encourage eating plans that cut out entire food groups. We want our members to be happy and enjoy the food they eat so we're not going to dictate what you should or shouldn't be consuming. We're all for having treats, especially if a slice of cake or glass of wine as a post-run reward motivates you to work up a sweat. But we're also aware that they have to be in moderation, and it is not recommended to overindulge in sugar, salt or alcohol.

While we're not going to tell you what you should be eating on the following pages, we do want to show how nutrition can play a part in your running performance and recovery, so you can then make an informed decision on what you choose to include in your diet.

On a day-to-day basis, the government recommends following a balanced diet via their NHS Eatwell Guide, and the recommended daily calorie intake for women is 2,000 (including those found in drinks). They advise having at least five portions of fruit or vegetables a day, either in the form of snacks or incorporated into main meals. They say a third of your daily intake should come from the fruit and vegetable category, and another third from starchy carbohydrates such as bread, rice, pasta, oats and potatoes. Eat wholegrain versions of bread, rice and pasta where possible as they have a lower glycaemic index (GI), which means they are broken down by the body to be used as energy at a slower rate. This means they will fuel you and make you feel fuller for longer, as opposed to high GI foods – such as potatoes and white bread – which will give a more instant but less prolonged boost to your energy levels. High GI foods do have a place in a runner's diet though. Having a high GI snack such as toasted white bread with jam or rice cakes shortly before a run means you can have a quick and easily-digested energy boost if you need something to keep you going within an hour of doing any exercise.

The Eatwell Guide also recommends that a fifth of your daily food intake comes from the protein category which includes things like fish, beans, pulses and eggs. Dairy (and alternative) products such as yoghurt, cheese and milk should be consumed in a similar amount but try to avoid versions that are high in sugar. They also recommend drinking six to eight 250 ml glasses of water a day and having only a very small amount of oils and spreads.

Outside their pie chart of recommended foods are those high in saturated fat and sugar, such as chocolate, cake, crisps, fizzy drinks, biscuits, sweets and ice cream. These are not recommended daily staples but can be enjoyed in moderation; after all, life would be pretty boring if we ate healthily all of the time and denied ourselves the odd treat. One of the joys of running is that you can indulge guilt-free as you'll be burning off some of the calories consumed.

PUT THE RIGHT FUEL IN YOUR TANK

While in general it is best to follow a healthy, balanced diet, runners sometimes have different requirements to meet the needs of the activity they are doing. We asked nutritionist Russ Best, a British elite athlete with numerous running accolades to his name – including winning the Royal Parks Half – to give us his expert advice (for more from Russ, visit his website www.simplyrussbest.me and follow him on Twitter at @SimplyRussBest).

When it comes to the best foods for runners to have before exercise, Best says: 'This ultimately comes down to two things: personal preference and effort. We all like to eat different things, and how we prepare and eat for running is no different. We need something we can stomach, literally, but we need to be mindful of what we're doing. The fuel required for an easy trot down the road differs from a long run or a hard hill session. If we're going hard (be honest!) we need sources of carbohydrate that are low in fibre such as a cereal bar, banana or the old-fashioned jam sandwich. If we're going for a long run we need to fuel up in advance, we'll need slower releasing, complex carbohydrates: porridge, jacket or sweet potatoes and a plateful of (wholemeal) pasta are all good options. Note these are slightly heavier on the stomach so give yourself more time to digest these. For up to an hour of easy running first thing, we don't necessarily need fuel, just some water or your morning cup of tea or coffee is enough.'

Many RMR members agree that, if they are just getting up and going for a short, easy early-morning run, they can do so without having breakfast first, as they will have adequate fuel in the tank from their evening meal the night before.

It's important to be mindful of what you eat before a run, as what you consume could not only affect your performance by giving you the energy to move, but also your enjoyment. You could find what you have eaten derails what could have been a good run if you make the mistake of opting for something that causes a stitch or runner's trots. If this does happen to you, think about what you ate beforehand and any changes you could make to avoid it happening in the future. Also consider the timing of when you eat your food before exercise. If you are having a large meal or something containing slow-release carbs, then allow at least two hours before working out to avoid a stitch or feeling sick. Some people even find they will need three to four hours. If you're having a snack of quick release energy like a banana, you should be okay to run within an hour.

EAT TO AID RECOVERY

Just as what we eat before a run can affect how we feel, what we eat afterwards is also important.

Protein is needed to help repair the muscle fibres damaged during exercise, so try to take some on within an hour of exercise, particularly if you've done a hard session, long run or race. Best says: 'Following exercise we need to think of the three Rs: Rehydrate, Refuel and Repair. To that end we need a source of fluid, a source of carbohydrate and a source of protein.'

Best says a glass of milk is the perfect solution because: 'A glass of full-fat cow's milk typically contains three point two grams of protein per one hundred millilitres, and four point eight grams of carbohydrate, along with reasonable amounts of vitamin B-12, vitamin D and calcium, so you can meet your protein and carbohydrate needs for repair and refuelling quite comfortably in one drink. More importantly, dairy is a complete protein, meaning it has a full complement of essential amino acids.'

Best says those watching their waistlines shouldn't be afraid of drinking full-fat milk as research has shown it is not the enemy of dieters despite its high fat content. However, if your personal preference is to have skimmed and semi-skimmed milks, these have similar levels of protein and carbs, so would also be appropriate post-race drinks.

But what if you can't drink milk because you are lactose-intolerant or vegan? Best says that if you have plant-based milks instead, soya is the best alternative as it is closest in protein content to cow's milk, whereas some nut milks only have half to a third of the amount of protein. To make the most of plant-based milks as a recovery drink, Best has the following advice: 'Plant milks are incomplete proteins meaning we would need to combine them with another food source to get all of our essential amino acids in. Practically speaking, cow's milk is nutritionally superior for athletes but if people prefer plant milks, opt for an unsweetened version that has been fortified with extra vitamins and minerals, and follow up with a meal containing all your essential amino acids. For vegetarians or vegans, this can be done by combining legumes, nuts, seeds and grains. For example, a bean chilli served with rice, topped with some toasted nuts for crunch would be a great post-session meal, or for something lighter a peanut butter sandwich is a quick fix.'

Chocolate-flavoured milk has also been proven to be beneficial after exercise because it is rehydrating and contains carbs, protein, salt and sugar. However, because the sugar content of flavoured milk is higher than in unflavoured milk, save the chocolate version for after hard sessions, races or long runs, rather than having it after every workout.

As well as cow's milk, nuts, fish, beans and eggs are also good sources of protein. Best says: 'Solid food options can be simple snacks such as a chicken salad wrap, a bowl of yoghurt with some fruit and muesli thrown on top or in winter months a simple, homemade vegetable and bean soup with some pasta or rice in the mix. Sushi is also an increasingly convenient option if you're travelling.'

By adequately refuelling after exercise you will be less likely to suffer from DOMS, so you won't be as achy in the days following a hard run. Not only will this make your daily activities more bearable, it will also mean you feel better on your next workout. Some find it more convenient to have protein shakes (drinks that can be mixed up using whey powder) and other processed high-protein snacks after a session where you have pushed yourself hard or a race. These kinds of products can aid your recovery, but you needn't worry about having them after every run as you should be able to refuel efficiently with what you can find in your kitchen cupboards and fridge, from a glass of milk to a boiled egg or handful of nuts.

FAB FOOD FOR RUNNERS

Here are some simple and satisfying foods that can aid your running and recovery.

▶ **Oats:** This really is the breakfast of champions! Oats make excellent running fuel as they are high in carbs, full of fibre and provide slow-release energy. They can also help lower cholesterol. You can keep it interesting by having oats as porridge or muesli and topping it with various nuts, seeds and fresh fruits for extra vitamins and minerals. You can also whizz some oats into smoothies or get oat cereal bars for a quick energy boost (but beware of ones excessively high in sugar).

▶**Milk:** As stated in the section on eating to aid recovery, cow's milk is the ultimate recovery drink as it contains protein and fat-soluble vitamins. It's also high in calcium which helps to make the bones stronger. If you have to have plant-based alternatives which aren't as high in protein, opt for unsweetened versions fortified with vitamins and minerals and consume them with another source of protein.

▶**Eggs:** Eggs are high in protein and vitamins and are quick and easy to cook so they make an excellent post-run meal or snack. They are also versatile – as you can scramble, boil, poach, fry or make an omelette with them, you won't get bored.

▶**Beetroot:** This vegetable has surged in popularity with runners in recent years after numerous studies have found it can enhance stamina and endurance. Another study found that eating a baked beetroot before a race can improve your speed. The secret to the vegetable's performance-enhancing powers is the fact that it's rich in nitrates. These compounds can increase the energy that's available to muscle cells. To get the benefits, drink beetroot juice regularly or incorporate it into meals, such as by adding it to salads or sandwiches, or having a beetroot risotto. Even better, how about disguising the flavour by occasionally making a beetroot chocolate cake? If you're not keen on beetroot, or the purple colour it can turn your urine, then you can get nitrates from other sources. Spinach, kale, rocket and other leafy green vegetables are also high in them, so add the green leaves to salads, smoothies, curries and sandwiches.

▶**Bananas:** While it is good to include lots of fruit in your daily diet, bananas are particularly good for runners as they contain quick-release carbs to fuel exercise. They are also high in potassium, which helps to maintain blood pressure, to strengthen your muscles and to regulate your body's fluid levels.

▶**Nuts:** A small portion of nuts can give you a large dose of vitamins and minerals, and they're also high in protein. A handful can make a quick snack to keep you going when you're working or if you're out and about, while having some after a run can aid recovery. They're easy to pack in your bag for after a race and eating a few nuts a day has been proven to be able to extend your life.

▶**Bread:** Bread contains carbs to fuel your exercise, and some varieties are fortified with extra iron and vitamins. In general, opt for wholemeal as this is broken down more slowly by the body and will provide you with energy for longer. White bread, on the other hand, is useful to have if you want a quick snack before running or racing as it contains quick-release carbs, and having it with jam will give you an extra boost. Bread is another product that is versatile and useful for both before and after running. Toast it, make a sandwich, dip it in a boiled egg or smother it in peanut butter.

TAKING SUPPLEMENTS

There are so many products on the shelves today promising to boost performance and aid recovery. The choice can be confusing and you might wonder if you need to take anything extra, whether in the form of a tablet or dissoluble powder. On the whole, you should be able to get all the nutrients you need to run and recover well by following a healthy, balanced diet with plenty of fruit and vegetables, carbs and protein as previously outlined.

However, there are some instances when taking a supplement could be beneficial. Best explains his position on whether it's necessary to take supplements: 'In a word no. In another, perhaps. Supplements should be supplementary to the body of the diet. Get the basics right consistently and your eating will serve your training well. Having said that, I often recommend athletes take fish oil or krill capsules (one to two grams per day) to help with overall health and if living in the UK, Europe or North America (i.e. countries where you might not have a lot of sunlight in certain seasons) I would also recommend a Vitamin D test to see if you are deficient and could benefit from upping your intake. Both of these supplements help keep athletes healthy, and a healthy athlete is a happy athlete. Vitamin C and Zinc are worth having in the cupboard to combat a cold. This killer combination can help cut cold duration by a day or so, allowing you to get back on track sooner!'

Meanwhile, women can benefit from other supplements depending on the current circumstances in their life. For instance, if you're pregnant, taking a folic acid supplement is recommended, and if you have heavy periods, taking on extra iron could help to boost energy levels.

Only ever take supplements made and sold by a reputable company, and be wary of anything making wild promises about how it might improve your athletic performance or change your body shape. If it sounds too good to be true, it probably is. Check the ingredients of any supplements you take and also research any side effects. Ensure you are actually deficient enough to warrant taking a supplement before you do so, as there can be consequences to overdosing on vitamins and minerals. For instance, excessive intake of iron can cause constipation, while overdosing on vitamin D can lead to kidney problems. If you are in any doubt whatsoever about taking a supplement, check with a medical professional first.

CARB-LOADING

When running a long-distance event like a marathon or an ultra, we have additional nutritional needs. Runners are advised to stock up on extra carbohydrates in the build-up to the event, known as carb-loading, so they have extra fuel for their muscles. Best explains why carb-loading is important: 'Increasing carbohydrate intake in the days leading up to a marathon boosts our muscle glycogen content. Glycogen is our muscle's preferred fuel source for intense activity (think of it as a big spiky ball made of sugar molecules), and stocking up your stores has been consistently shown to improve race performance. Two to three days out from your marathon, increase your carbohydrate and decrease your fibre intake. Rice, bread, breakfast cereals and fruit smoothies are good sources of carbohydrate in the final build-up. My pre-race go-to is a risotto, but a mild curry (as long as you have had this before a race before so you know it agrees with you and don't choose anything too spicy) or a pizza are always easy to get hold of if you're away from home the night before your race.'

Bread, pasta, potatoes, pulses and beans are all good sources of carbs for when you are looking to boost your intake before a long race. Up the frequency of when you eat these foods three days out from the race, for example, by having meals as well as snacks high in carbs, rather than just increasing your mealtime portions of the food. This way, you won't end up feeling too stuffed and bloated from one sitting.

Carb-loading before a marathon can prevent you from 'hitting the wall' during the race as you will be less likely to become depleted of energy if your glycogen stores are topped up. However, there is a limit to these stores and, as the marathon distance is such a long way, they will be used up before you reach the finish. This is why you also need to top up by consuming carbs on the run. In a half and a marathon you can do this via energy gels and drinks. Sweets, such as jelly babies, are also favoured by some runners for a quick boost. Whichever product you intend to take on race day, you need to practise consuming it beforehand to ensure it agrees with you. Some find certain products can give them stomach ache or runner's trots. As a result, don't take any snacks, such as jelly sweets, that are being handed out by well-meaning members of the crowd unless you already know they won't adversely affect your run. Best explains: 'I would recommend "training your gut" from at least six weeks before your big race. Long runs are a great place to practise this — try one gel or a couple of your favourite gummy sweets every thirty to forty-five minutes. Practise eating (and drinking) as you run as this will get you used to managing your feeding when on the move, saving a lot of panic on race day and avoiding becoming a sticky mess!'

However, Best recommends only practising taking on energy gels and drinks on your weekly long run, and not on every run. 'Most of your training should be completed without these products; this keeps you burning fat as fuel, and decreases your reliance on the products,' he says.

For those running an ultra, you'll need to take on even more carbs as you go along in order to complete the long distance. Food might be provided at checkpoints along the way, but you should also carry energy gels and drinks and some easy-to-digest snacks such as rice cakes and flapjacks so you always have something when you need it. Once again, it is important to practice what you eat in training so you know what works for you.

Remember, your carb stores only become depleted when you are running long distances, so carb-loading in the days leading up to a short race such as a 5k or 10k is not necessary. Instead, just have a pre-race evening meal containing some carbs (read on for suggestions from RMR members) and a good breakfast, such as porridge or toast.

STAYING HYDRATED

Throughout the book, the importance of staying hydrated in order to run well has been frequently mentioned. If you become dehydrated on a run you can become nauseous and light-headed and struggle to keep going. You might develop cramp, or feel like you don't have the energy to go on. However, there are also consequences to drinking too much, so don't go overboard. Too much liquid before a run could give you a stitch and make you desperate to use the toilet. In extreme cases, excessive consumption of water can cause hyponatremia, a condition that, in rare cases, can be fatal because it flushes salt from the body and makes the brain swell.

In general, using common sense will enable you to drink adequately. Unless it is a particularly hot day, when you're doing a short, easy run you shouldn't need to laden yourself down with water bottles – just have a glass of water before you go and another (and/or a glass of milk) on your return. If it's hot or humid, you'll need to drink extra as you'll be losing more fluid due to sweating more. If you are going for a long run of an hour or more, pushing yourself doing intervals, doing a tempo run or if you're racing you'll need to drink more than you would on a short, easy run because the extra effort will make you sweat more. How much you sweat will also depend on your genes and build, so don't compare how much you drink to others – work out what is best for you.

A simple way to learn how hydrated you are is to regularly check the colour of your urine. If it is a dark brown or orange shade, this is a sign you are dehydrated and need to up your liquid intake. The clearer the wee is, the more hydrated you are. How frequently you need to go to the toilet is also an indication: if you haven't needed to go for hours, it's likely you're not drinking enough. Remember that hot drinks also count towards your daily fluid intake. It's a myth that tea and coffee are dehydrating, but bear in mind that they can make you need the toilet more as they are diuretic, so it might not be wise to have too many cups before running or racing.

There are additional benefits to having caffeine before exercise: it has been proven to enhance athletic performance as it can improve endurance. It is also a stimulant, so it can make your body and mind feel more alert. However, once again moderation is key, as too much caffeine is not good for us.

When it comes to drinking on the run, as stated previously, you should only need to do so when covering long distances, when working hard (for example, racing) and on particularly hot days. On long training runs, you'll need to carry your own water. If you don't like to carry a bottle in your hand you can get belts and hydration backpacks to make this easier. You could also hide a bottle along your route the day before a long run, or, if you're running out and back again the same way, drop it off somewhere on the way out and pick it up again on your return.

At most races, there will be manned water stations providing water to drink along the course. It can be a fine art to be able to drink and run at the same time, particularly if you are handed water in a cup rather than a bottle, so you might want to practise this in training if you are going for a PB, as you don't want to lose time in the race by stopping to sip your drink. Squeezing the cup to create a funnel can help ensure that more water goes in your mouth than down your front as you try to drink on the move. Some water stations in large-participation races can become congested, so be careful not to cut up a fellow competitor as you dive for a drink. Also be aware of where you throw any discarded bottles or cups and make sure that they don't trip up runners behind you.

Drinking frequently during a long-distance run or a race like a half, a marathon or an ultra is particularly important. The key is to not drink excessive amounts in one go but to drink little and often, starting at three to five miles into the race. If you leave it till you feel thirsty, you might already be dehydrated. Remember that if it's hot and sunny on race day you will need to drink more than usual.

RMR MEMBERS REVEAL THEIR FAVOURITE PRE- AND POST-RACE MEALS

Not sure what to eat before a race to help you run well, or what to have after to aid recovery? Of course everyone is different but here some of our RMR members reveal what works for them to give you some ideas.

The night before:

'Pizza! I always have pizza the night before a morning race.'
Shontelle Jones

'Marathon burritos (rice, tomatoes, beans and spices in wholemeal tortilla wraps, full recipe available at www.bbcgoodfood.com).'
Helen Brant

'Homemade pizza. With loads of veggies and cheese then rocket on top (after it's cooked). It's got me round London and numerous halfs.'
Kitty Tompsett

'Spaghetti Bolognese.'
Fiona Sawkill

'Pasta with chicken and broccoli cooked in a creamy cheese sauce – my hubby makes it and it's soooo good!'
Louise Milward-Lawson

'*Either paella or pizza.*'
Rosie Bassett

'*Chicken and chorizo pasta bake, nom nom nom!*'
Vicky Pollington

'*My pre-race meal is chicken and mushroom risotto.*'
Clair Ramsden

'*My pre-race meal is almost always leek and bacon risotto, scrummy yummy.*'
Tracey Francis

'*Pasta, cheese and beans the night before, or special chow mein.*'
Kelly Reeves

'*Spaghetti Bolognese the night before, usually. Although sometimes it's something like steak and chips. I'm also mindful in the whole week before the race of eating well and drinking enough water.*'
Jenni Johnston

The morning of the run...

'I always have porridge with cinnamon and honey for brekkie.'
Shirley Storey

*'Pre morning-race meal is simple for me –
a slice of toast and jam, or a banana.'*
Claire Wilson

'I have white toast and jam.'
Georgina Walker

*'Morning of the race – scrambled eggs on toast.
It keeps me filled up.'*
Jenni Johnston

After the race...

*'It has to be chocolate milk. It's amazing and tastes so good
whatever the weather and whatever the run.'*
Tamie Slade

'After a long run I love peanut butter and banana on toast.'
Donna McAllister

'*Post-race is always bacon, egg and avocado or I make a smoothie by mixing vanilla-flavour protein powder with 300 ml almond milk, nut butter, raspberries and mango and zero per cent fat yoghurt.*'

Vicky Pollington

RMR RECOMMENDED RECIPES

These simple and easy recipes as tried and tested by RMR members will help you pre and post run.

▶**Leanne Davies's three berry smoothie:** A few strawberries, raspberries and blackberries (frozen make the smoothie lovely and chilled), 2 tbsp natural yoghurt, 200 ml milk, 100 ml water (add 1 tsp honey if you need a natural sugar) whizz up – done!

▶**Danielle Wilson's pre-run breakfast:** One mashed banana mixed with a whisked egg, a dessert spoon of peanut butter and a dessert spoon of oats. Dollop a few spoonfuls in a frying pan and cook for a few minutes each side to get drop scones/American pancakes.

▶**Lucy Waterlow's post-run banana milkshake:** One banana, a glass of milk and a small pinch of cinnamon. Whizz in a blender and voila! The milk will hydrate you and has protein to aid muscle repair, bananas contain carbs and vitamins while cinnamon has anti-inflammatory properties.

If you make this with a plant-based milk, blend in a few chia seeds to increase the protein, as plant-based milks don't contain as much protein as cow's milk.

▶ **Bunty Rance's post-run smoothie:** Blend a banana, a handful of spinach and a few pineapple pieces with a glass of almond milk and a teaspoon of coconut-flavoured whey protein. It's a non-alcoholic piña colada!

▶ **Philly Williamson's oat energy bars:** Mash up two over-ripe bananas with 120 ml vegetable oil and 110 g sugar. In another bowl mix up dry ingredients of 135 g oats, 95 g plain flour and 1 tsp baking powder, with a few drops of vanilla extract, a pinch of salt and ½ tsp cinnamon and ½ tsp nutmeg. Combine this mixture with the mashed banana and then mix in 95 g walnuts and 75 g cranberries (note: you can mix and match what nuts and fruits you use and also add seeds – the choice is yours). Spread the mixture evenly in a greased baking tray and cook at gas mark 4/180°C for around fifteen minutes, or until a skewer comes out clean. Cut into squares and enjoy!

For more on discussing healthy eating with our members, join our subgroup, The Healthier Balance, via the RMR Facebook group.

CHAPTER SEVEN:
PAY IT FORWARD

At RMR, we believe kindness is everything. That's why you won't find any criticism or negative comments about other women in the posts on our pages, and why so many of our members feel safe enough to share their running concerns and problems with one another: they know they will always be met with support. We want this ethos to spread beyond our Facebook page to our running community and the wider world. We know we are not going to be able to achieve world peace, but we can still make a difference to the lives of others in small but significant ways. One of the easiest ways to do this is to always greet fellow runners with a friendly smile or word of encouragement, whether you are passing them by on your own run, watching them in a race or training in the same group. Never underestimate what a warm smile and an atmosphere of positivity can do to boost someone else's spirit.

We encourage those who have discovered a love of running – and all the happiness and confidence it brings – to 'pay it forward' by helping others to get into the sport and to enable them to overcome any barriers that may have prevented them exercising before. RMR's Jennifer McLarnon said that the support of faster runners has made such a difference to her in her quest to get fitter. She said: 'My bestest running mate, Leesa Pethick, is paying it forward in an amazing way. She was a beginner and remembers how hard it was to come last in races. She has supported me through a number of races and makes sure I'm not last by ducking back and coming in behind me! During my first 10k, she and two other lovely ladies in my running club (Plymouth Harriers, the best running family ever) joined me so I knew I wasn't alone and they stuck with me all the way. I see her giving up her race to support me as the ultimate support, and I can't wait to find my person to pay it forward to when I get faster.'

Being friendly and welcoming is particularly important when it comes to new members joining your running club. For many, it can take a great deal of courage to go along to a club training session for the first time. Some might feel they aren't 'good' enough to be there and may be worried they will be left behind. If you see someone who looks apprehensive or nervous at your club then always make them feel welcome. Some clubs will have a set-up to make things easier for new recruits – such as a buddy system or designated training nights for new members – or have appointed someone whose role it is to welcome newbies and help them settle in.

If your club doesn't have anything like this in place, perhaps you could volunteer to help out in such a capacity, or speak to whoever runs the club or its committee about things they could do to make joining up easier for apprehensive novices. Remember: most running clubs are run by volunteers who give up their time freely to support runners and to help others get into the sport. Find out if you can help too. There are often various roles available within running clubs that need willing and able volunteers, from coaching to updating the club's website to organising social activities for members.

SET UP YOUR OWN RUNNING GROUP

If you don't have a running club in your area that adequately caters for beginners, or if you would like to do something to help others start running, why not set up your own group? One of the best ways to do this is to get a Leadership In Running Fitness (LiRF) qualification from England Athletics. Their one-day courses, held around the country, qualify and insure participants to lead runs. England Athletics say of the course: 'It will enable you to deliver fun and safe sessions to multi-ability groups and give advice and support to the new runner, as well as developing pathways for those who want to progress. It focuses on understanding and overcoming barriers to participation in running and how to increase participation by those not traditionally attracted to a running club.' At the time of writing, the course costs £160 (reduced to £140 for England Athletics affiliated club members) and it is a legal requirement that you have a DBS check with UK Athletics. Some established clubs may agree to pay for your course if you will lead group runs for their members afterwards. Some workplaces may also pay for you to do it if you can help employees to get fit. RMR's Jo Gennari became a run leader for her colleagues and the group she set up has been a hit. She said: 'I work in a London NHS Hospital Trust and I did my LiRF last year at the request of my workplace wellbeing group. I then helped lead one beginners' group through the C25K, meeting one evening a week for twelve weeks (follow us on Twitter @LGT_Runners). It was such a success that all members of the group expressed a wish to continue training together after completing the plan to work on improving their distances and speeds further. We intend to field a large team in the Big Half in London next March and to get another group to follow the C25K plan. As well as helping members of staff get fit and gain in running confidence, many said they enjoyed the increased interaction with colleagues that they didn't normally work with.'

Following the LiRF, further qualifications, such as Coach In Running Fitness (CiRF), can then be gained if you want to expand your knowledge and services. For more information, visit www.englandathletics.org. There are also a number of businesses that train up group leaders to deliver running classes. If you run your group through an already established company, they might be able to support you with advertising and offer you further coaching advice. However, if you prefer to strike out on your own and set up your own group instead, then the advantages are that you can call the shots – where and when your group will meet, and whether you will charge participants to attend. It will then be down to you to advertise your group and support your members. You might decide to organise something free and more informal and just arrange for groups of friends to meet regularly, or you could volunteer to take group runs and training sessions for your athletics club. You could also start a running club for children if you want to get young people active.

A number of RMR members have set up their own running groups and found it highly rewarding. One of them is Emma Talbot, who said: 'I completed the Leadership in Running Fitness course, pulled my big-girl pants up so high they tucked into my bra, roped in some friends and went for it! Eight months later, one hundred and fifty-five women have been through our beginners' programme and thirty to forty women regularly turn out for our group runs.' Find out more about Emma's group at www.icanrunclub.co.uk.

Another who helped found a club is Jodie Evans. She said: 'I helped set up a running group with friends called Cwmbran Pub Runners (www.cwmbranpubrunners.co.uk). We completed the C25K with a local running group and felt we wanted to carry on running but with an emphasis on fun rather than being competitive. Our coach from the C25K group, Jo Everson, said she would take a few of us for runs and organised the routes. Word spread and she named the group so it was clear we were a social group and not a 'serious' one – although we take our medals seriously! Jo set up a Facebook page and website and word got around so we now have around sixty members. There is no pressure, and to join us is free. We all take part in events and have regular nights out. It's a club for all and works really well.'

She adds: 'My advice to anyone looking to start their own running group is to begin with a few friends and all talk about it, showing how enthusiastic you are. Word will soon get around. Have a Facebook page to direct people and it will grow! We also get loads of interest when we wear our tops at events and parkrun.'

RMR STORIES

Kate Glascott, 36, and Bianca Pridham, 34, from Wells, Somerset, decided to 'pay it forward' by helping more people discover a love of running and make new friendships, just like they did.

Kate says...

As I watched people who I'd helped complete the C25K plan celebrate finishing their first 5K, I was overwhelmed with a feeling of pride and accomplishment. In some ways it felt even better than when I had finished the plan myself! It had been amazing to help them achieve something they thought they could never do.

Three years before this, I was a person who always avoided exercise and I had a constant battle with my weight. I had always wanted to be able to run but, despite a few lone attempts, had failed miserably. When my local running club, Wells City Harriers, set up a new group called Up and Running, which would follow the C25K plan, I decided to give it another try. Bianca and I met each other at the first training session and we supported one another every step of the way. Yes, it was hard at times, but we stuck together and helped each other through it. I still remember that feeling of amazement at the end of each week when we realised how far we had come, like the first time we ran non-stop for a certain amount of time, or when we had accomplished a mile – something I personally never thought was achievable. We had a lovely group, and after running the 5k Wells Fun Run at the end of the course we decided to stick with it and carry on running with the club. I'm now toned and can't believe I can actually call myself fit! When the Harriers decided to do the 'Up and Running' course again the following year, I was more than happy to help out. I had gone from being someone who avoided exercise to enjoying it, and I wanted to help others do the same.

Last year, the Harriers asked Bianca and I if we would like to become Run Leaders so we could take a greater role in their latest Up and Running initiative. We said yes immediately as we thought it would be a wonderful way to 'pay it forward'. We completed the LiRF course, so we were qualified and insured, and then led a group along with two of our original coaches. The participants varied from those who had never run before to those returning to the sport after a long time away. It was so rewarding to see them improve and complete the Wells Fun Run, just like we had three years before. Bianca and I have carried on as Run Leaders for the club's beginners' group, which has now grown from fewer than ten people to over 30 people in just one year. We love it – we wouldn't miss our Wednesday evening sessions for the world!

Bianca says...

In a similar way to Kate, I had tried running on my own, or with friends and family many times before and had always given up. I always felt I wasn't good enough. In 2012, after I had my youngest daughter, I experienced post-natal depression. I lost three stone due to ill health and my marriage breaking down. I was the slim person I had always wanted to be but the unhappiest I had ever been. I didn't live near family and I didn't have many friends nearby as we had moved for work reasons before starting a family.

By 2013 I had begun a new life. I was happier and started to gain some weight again. I had a new partner who was very active and we both loved being outdoors, so I was motivated to get fitter. When I saw an advert for the Up and Running course my partner pretty much kicked me out of the door, telling me that I would be fine and that I should just go and try it. Attending the first session I was so nervous, and I had no idea what to expect. But I soon discovered that the group was fantastic, the course was perfectly paced and the sense of achievement was amazing, week after week. It was hard some weeks – I didn't think I could do it, but I did. For the first time since moving to Somerset I had friends like Kate who weren't linked to my children or work. I can't emphasise enough the impact the group has had on my running, my social life and wellbeing. Running makes me so happy!

It was great to be able to offer support the following year. The small groups allowed a more bespoke, individual course to be offered and for many more abilities to take part than in the previous year. It was eye-opening to see how far I had come – now people were asking me for advice, I was a runner! I discovered I enjoyed leading and encouraging others – I loved seeing them develop. When they crossed a finishing line or achieved a PB, I felt as proud as when I had done it.

I think the Harrier's coaches saw that Kate and I were normal people who love to run, which is just what people need to see when they turn up to a new club or group, so they asked us to be Run Leaders. We aren't really fast – we drink wine and eat cake! But we love to see others achieve what they didn't think they could. We love to share our enthusiasm for running (which is one of the reasons we also love RMR) and even in the winter we have often have more than 20 people turning up for our group run on a Wednesday night, where no one is left behind. I would like to think that, along with the coaches, Kate and I are one of the reasons that numbers continue to grow, people turn up week after week and they continue to love to run. I'm so proud of what we have achieved, and I hope we can continue to help many more discover a love of running like we have.

GIVE BACK BY VOLUNTEERING

Another way to give something back to the running community is by volunteering to help out at a race. There are often various roles available, from marshalling to handing out water, but each one is important and vital for the smooth running of the race. Many events, particularly parkruns, can only take place thanks to those who give up their time for free. Marshals, especially, are imperative at races to ensure the runners' safety. They might have to stand on the same spot for hours to direct participants on the correct route, control traffic flow and just generally encourage weary runners to keep going (and to organise first aid if they get into difficulty). If you're racing yourself, always listen to the instructions from marshals and be grateful to them for putting themselves out so you can enjoy a race in safety. Volunteering to be a marshal means you can give something back if you race regularly. It can be tiring to stand around for hours, and not always much fun, especially if it's a cold and wet day, but it is rewarding, and watching and encouraging others could motivate you in your own endeavours.

parkrun are in need of volunteers every week to ensure the 5k runs can take place. As well as marshals, they need people to do various other jobs such as timing the runs, scanning barcodes at the finish, collating the results and being the tail runner/walker to ensure no participant is left behind. It was once thought that parkrun could never be successful because it would rely on so many people giving up their time for free on Saturday mornings to make it happen. But the thousands who do so every week prove how supportive and selfless the running community can be.

If you participate regularly in parkrun then why not give something back by volunteering a couple of times a year at your local event or junior equivalent? It's a great way to stay involved if you can't currently run too, for instance, if you're recovering from a race or an injury. You can take the children along to help out as well. RMR's Jessamy Carlson became a Run Director for her local junior parkrun after she took up running three years ago following a health scare. Her role involves overseeing the event by briefing the volunteers, helping to set up and dismantle the course and giving instructions to the participants at the start. She says she loves how the role allows her to boost her health and that of her children, as well as helping other families enjoy running. She says: 'I was determined to make running and exercise part of my life. I'm proud to inspire my four-year-old who wants to "run like Mummy".'

If there isn't a parkrun or junior parkrun in your area, another way to give something back to the running community is to set one up yourself. RMR's Ellen Williams helped set up the Cannock Chase parkrun in Staffordshire and has the following advice: 'The things you need before thinking about setting up a parkrun are: a really reliable and enthusiastic team of volunteers (you will need to call on these week in and week out over the first few weeks and even months), funding (approximately two thousand five hundred pounds) and a suitable location. I was a member of one of four local running clubs invited to help set up a parkrun at Cannock Chase: Chase Harriers, Chasewater Runners, Rugeley Runners and Stafford Harriers. We were fortunate in that we had all of these boxes ticked – Staffordshire County Council wanted a parkrun in the middle of the borough so they gave permission for the use of the land, and they were also able to fund the venture.

'Once you (and parkrun) have agreed that you are definitely going to be setting up an event, you need to identify one or two Event Directors, two Run Directors and about twelve named volunteers in order to show support for the venture. Paperwork needs to be filled out and everything needs approving by parkrun – risk assessments, emergency procedures, etc. You then need to finalise, measure and have approved by your ambassador (who parkrun will put you in touch with) a suitable route. There are lots of things to bear in mind when thinking about the route, such as avoiding downhill finishes and minimising the number of laps to ensure there aren't issues arising from the range of speeds of runners. Your parkrun ambassador holds your hand through the whole process so you and your "core team" will be in good hands! Our first parkrun was huge, with five hundred and sixty-nine runners turning up! The people of Staffordshire had apparently been long awaiting a parkrun in the beauty spot that is Cannock Chase.

'Setting up a parkrun is hard work but without a doubt it is one of the most rewarding experiences I have ever had the opportunity to be involved with. It was a whole team effort by the four local running clubs and we had complete support from the Rangers at Staffordshire County Council. There is no greater feeling than seeing the happy, sweaty, smiley faces of walkers and runners from all walks of life coming together to enjoy a timed run on a Saturday morning, in the company of friends or strangers who become friends... and knowing that you were one of the people that helped set up that parkrun!'

Visit www.parkrun.com for more information on how you can volunteer or set up your own event.

MAKE SOME NOISE AT RACES

You will have noticed in chapter five on racing (page 142) that many of the RMR runners loved certain events because of the atmosphere, and that is created by people like you! If you are going along to watch then make as much noise as you can. Your energy could really lift a runner when they are struggling. Bang a tambourine, blow a whistle or just clap and whoop. Make a banner with an inspiring or amusing slogan, or offer to give runners a high five or free sweets such as jelly babies. Shout positive and encouraging words like 'You look strong!' or 'Great running, you can do it!' Try to avoid telling a runner they are 'nearly there' unless they are within 400 m of the finish line though, as otherwise they might not thank you for it!

RMR members say the support of strangers can really elevate them when they are tiring in a race. Sara Tamsin Richards says: 'The most encouraging words I had at the London Marathon were from a guy in the crowd who looked me straight in the eye and said "You're looking great Tamsin, you've got this, you know you can do it, keep going." I won't forget his words of encouragement for a very long time.' Deborah Bullingham adds: 'The most encouraging thing people can say, in my experience, is "You've got this." The least useful is "keep running" or "nearly there" – someone shouted it to me at mile five of the London Marathon and I wanted to kill them! My all-time favourite was "You can still win this", which just made me chuckle.'

Pick out the names of runners to cheer on individually if they have written them on their vests, or single them out via their club name or race number. Save extra-loud cheers for anyone you see racing in RMR kit! RMR's Lisa Stevens said that this has made a big difference to her when racing. She says: 'The best supporters cheer you whether you're first or last with equal enthusiasm. Little kids collecting high fives always encourage me too. When your name is on your number and people take the time to cheer you on personally – that's extra encouraging. Or when I'm wearing RMR gear and someone yells "Run mummy run".'

RMR's Louise Spinney said a number of banners she's spotted at races have made her smile. She says: 'Signs that make you laugh are good. I've laughed when I've seen "Smile if you need the toilet" and "If Trump can run America, you can run 26.2 miles." I don't appreciate "nearly there" signs, as telling me that I have four miles left to go in a marathon is not nearly there!' She adds that when it comes to handing out sweets, always unwrap them first if they are of an individually wrapped variety so that the runner can easily grab and eat them on the go. Maxine Sinda Napal adds that handing out crisps also goes down well in her experience. She says: 'A friend recently held out a bag of salty crisps at mile twenty-two of the London Marathon and people swarmed on it! At that point you're needing a bit of salt, so having salty snacks on offer late in the race is very welcome.' Others say slices of satsuma and oranges have been greatly appreciated when handed to them by members of the crowd in races.

RMR often organise cheer squads at races so members can meet up and celebrate the achievements of those taking part. Knowing that the friendly bunch will be at a certain point to offer hugs, high fives and encouragement can really motivate and help runners to keep going. Come and join us!

FUNDRAISING TIPS FOR SUPPORTING CHARITIES THROUGH RACING

Running is a wonderful way to raise money for good causes. Many charities offer places in coveted races such as the London

Marathon in return for raising money via sponsorship. You could also take it upon yourself to do a particularly hard event or to take part in a race in fancy dress to raise awareness and funds for a cause close to your heart.

However, if you want to raise as much money as possible, or reach a target set by a charity in order to race for them, it can be difficult, particularly if you don't want to keep asking the same friends, family and colleagues for money. There are lots of other ways you can boost your charity coffers though. Setting up a way for people to sponsor you online is the easiest way for people to donate and you can share the address on your social media pages. RMR's Sandra Rhodes has an ingenious tip for maximising awareness of your charity page. She said: 'I added my sponsorship link to the bottom of my home and work emails (make sure your employer is okay with the work one). JustGiving have an app that allows you to include a "donate now" button and it also worked well for me.'

Other RMR members have held various events or found fun ways for friends and family to help them reach their targets. Here are a few fundraising ideas they recommend.

▶ **Host a coffee morning or afternoon tea:** Invite guests and ask them to make a donation to attend, then tuck into delicious treats while sharing a hot drink with good company. In the spring and summer, you could also host a picnic or barbecue.

▶ **Hold a quiz night:** Who doesn't enjoy a good quiz? Charge teams to enter and set some brainteasers for them to ponder. They'll have fun and might learn something too.

▶**Organise a raffle:** Sara Tamsin Richards has had success raising money this way. She says: 'Raffles are great – local businesses will donate prizes so don't be afraid to ask (for example, you could see if a local hairdresser could offer a free cut as a prize) and local attractions might happily give free tickets to events.'

▶**Go to a car-boot or table-top sale:** As they say, one person's junk is another's treasure. This option could declutter your home, raise extra money for your charity and give new life to an item you've not been making use of.

▶**Supermarket bag pack:** Ask your local store if you can pack bags for their customers for a day in return for them making a donation.

▶**School non-uniform day:** If you're a teacher or have a child of school age, see if the school will allow pupils to have a non-uniform day in return for donating money to your cause. You could do a similar thing in your workplace with a 'dress down' or fancy dress day.

▶**Cake sales:** Make some cakes and then sell them one lunch hour at work, at your local parkrun or in your child's playground if the school will allow it. You should make a good profit by charging per slice or cupcake and we bet you won't have any leftovers. Karen Bircham said that this worked well for her when she organised a cake sale for her colleagues. She said: 'I'm a teacher and my best fundraising idea has been a cake sale for staff over two days. Staff donated cakes and then everyone donated money to eat them. I raised eighty-five pounds from people just eating cake at work and it was zero effort to organise apart from a group email asking for donations.'

Meanwhile, Deborah Bullingham said that she had similar success when she sold ice creams: 'I'm a teacher too and the easiest money I raised for my charity was selling ice creams at the end of term in the playground. I did vanilla cones with a flake and sauce for one pound and raised two hundred and twenty in the space of about twenty minutes. I got my colleagues to pitch in and we had a production line going.' In another cake themed-tip, Sheila Rodenhurst recommends creating a delicious showstopper and then giving people the chance to win it as a prize. She said: 'If you can, bake a cake, then fill a piece of card with squares (I did fifty) and sell each square for a pound. A winning square is then picked and the person who bought that square gets the cake – and you get an easy fifty pounds for your charity.'

▶ **Dog walking:** Offer to walk the pets of friends, family and neighbours for a donation.

▶ **Sell each mile:** This works better the longer the race you are doing! Jodie Evans, who has raised money for charity this way, explains: 'I sold each mile of the marathon for twenty pounds and placed the names of those who had sponsored each mile on my top.'

▶ **Collect small change:** It's amazing how much small change can add up. Give friends and relatives a Smarties tube or similar and ask them to fill it with 20 pence pieces. Alternatively, ask them to keep filling it for you with the little coins like five and ten pence pieces they hate carrying around in their purses.

▶ **Organise a servant auction:** Get some willing volunteers and then auction them off to the highest bidder to do their household chores and cooking for a day.

▶ **Hold a lottery:** Sell the numbers and pick a date to draw a number at random. The person with the winning number takes a percentage of your takings, and you give the rest to your charity.

▶ **Place your bets:** Organise a sweepstake where friends and relatives can pay to make a guess at your finishing time or position. The closest to the actual result gets a percentage of the takings and you keep the rest for charity. Denise Taylor said that this made fundraising more fun for her and her friends. She says: 'I hate continually asking for sponsor money. When I ran for The Stroke Association this year they included a sheet for a sweepstake on race finish time. Friends at my running club and elsewhere enjoyed guessing how long I'd take to do the 10k, and one of them won twenty-five pounds.'

▶ **Have a bingo night:** Friends will enjoy taking part and can make a donation to get involved.

▶ **Pay for pampering:** If you have the skill, you could charge friends for manicures, pedicures and massages. If you don't, consider hiring someone who does to do it for you – as long as they agree to give a percentage of what they earn to your charity. You could employ a hairdresser to do cuts and styling, for example.

▶ **Have an open garden:** Got an outdoor space that you are particularly proud of and lots of beautiful plants, trees and flowers to show off? Organise an open garden and charge a fee for guests to come and see your green-fingered accomplishments.

▶ **Grow your own veggies:** Start up a vegetable patch and, once it is flourishing, ask for donations in return for people enjoying the fruits of your labour.

▶ **Car wash:** Grab a bucket and sponge and charge friends and family for your services to make their cars spotless for them.

▶ *Come Dine With Me*: Get friends to join you in replicating the Channel 4 show by having meals at one another's homes and rating one another's efforts, all in good spirit of course. You'll get to eat some tasty meals, enjoy time with friends and raise money at the same time by asking them all to make a donation to get involved.

▶ **Babysit:** Offer to give fellow mums a night out by babysitting in return for a charity donation.

►**Get crafty:** If you are artistic, create personalised keepsakes or drawings of friends' pets and children in return for a donation.

►**Put on a show:** If you have a talent for playing a musical instrument or singing, organise a performance and sell tickets for people to come and watch. If you think you have what it takes to make people laugh, you could do your own stand-up gig.

►**Get publicity:** Contact your local newspaper and tell them of your plans to run and any fundraising events you are organising to drum up interest and raise awareness.

►**Write a blog or regularly update your social media accounts:** Sharing the highs and lows of your training could prompt people to dig deep when they see how hard you're working to achieve your goal. Ali Masterson said she found this beneficial. She said: 'I recently did the Vitality London 10k and managed to raise one thousand pounds for my chosen local charity. I used JustGiving and made sure I updated my page every week with photos and how my training was going. I used Twitter, Facebook and Instagram to raise my profile and my firm also supported me and re-tweeted my sponsorship details. I talked about all the stuff that I was struggling with in training. I think I'm such an unlikely runner that people sponsored me out of sheer shock that I was running any further than the pub!'

▶ **Time your event with a milestone birthday:** Then you can ask those who might usually buy you a card or present to donate the money to your charity instead.

▶ **'Put your money where your miles are':** This strategy was adopted by Maxine Sinda Napal who explains: 'For my last Race For Life Half I donated fifty pence per mile I trained. I also dedicated every mile to someone who was fighting, or has sadly lost, their battle with cancer and asked friends to give me the names of loved ones. Then I donated a monetary amount in that person's name, equal to the time it took me to run the mile, so an eleven-minute fifteen-second mile was eleven pounds and fifteen pence, etc. When I made those personal donations, I asked people to match the amounts. Donating eleven pounds and fifteen pence doesn't hit the pocketbook as hard as twenty pounds and up, so it encouraged people to donate.'

RMR GLOSSARY

Are you confused by tempo runs and baffled by fartleks? Unsure what some members mean when they complain about cockwombles or say they 'Jeffed' a marathon? Then here is our handy Run Mummy Run Glossary, an A–Z guide of common running terms, acronyms and abbreviations.

▶ **Active recovery:** Low-intensity exercise such as swimming and walking that can help your body recover from a hard running session or race.

▶ **Age grading:** This figure is often given as a percentage in race results. It compares your performance to others based on your age and gender. The higher the percentage, the better you have performed.

▶ **Arm sleeves/warmers:** Worn by runners who want to keep their arms warm when the weather is a bit chilly without over-heating in a long-sleeved top. The fabric covers the upper arm and forearm.

▶ **Aqua-jogging**: Running in a swimming pool. This is often done when injured to maintain some fitness without putting any stress on the joints. You need to wear a special float around the waist to keep you upright so you can run in the water.

▶ **Barefoot running**: Running without shoes on. Some believe we were born to run this way and that exercising without bulky trainers reduces the chance of injury. Alternatively you can get 'barefoot' trainers, which have no cushioning but offer some protection from stepping on stones etc.

▶ **Bib (for racing)**: Another word for the number you pin to your vest in a race.

▶ **Blowing up/bonking**: A phrase used to explain why you didn't race as well as you'd hoped. Runners usually 'blow up' in a race if they have gone off too fast because they struggle to keep their pace going and get slower and feel worse as the race goes on.

▶ **Buggy running**: A popular way for new parents to run with their baby. Specialist running buggies have been designed to keep your baby safe and to make running comfortable for you. For more information about buggy running see chapter one, page 30.

▶ **Cadence:** Referring to running technique, your cadence is how many times your foot strikes the ground in one minute of running. The ideal is thought to be 180 foot strikes per minute, but this can vary depending on your pace and height. Improving your cadence can help you run more efficiently and could reduce your risk of injury. You can enhance your cadence by avoiding overstriding – aim for your foot to land under your hip instead of far in front of it.

▶ **Carb-loading:** This is what runners traditionally do before long-distance races, such as half marathons and marathons, to ensure they have enough fuel to run. Carbs are the body's main source of energy and are broken down into sugars by the digestive system to make the muscles and organs work. If it is not needed at the time of consumption, it is stored as glycogen. Carb-loading ensures that these glycogen stores are fully topped up before a long-distance run. Read more about carb-loading in chapter six, page 211.

▶ **Chip time:** Your exact race time as recorded by a chip if the race makes use of such technology.

Chips are sometimes incorporated into your race number, or they can be a tag that you attach to your laces or tie around your ankle. The chip will be activated when you pass over a mat on the start line and will accurately record your time until you cross another mat at the finish.

▶ **CiRF:** Abbreviation of Coach in Running Fitness, a course run by UK Athletics (UKA). Normally completed after the Leader in Running Fitness course (LiRF). Successful completion of the course means you receive your UKA coaching licence. If you are looking for a running coach it's worth checking that they have this qualification.

▶ **Cockwomble, also CW:** This is a term used by RMR members to describe an unsupportive partner. They might undermine your running or make it difficult for you to train and race. Also see frockwomble.

▶ **Compression socks:** Tightly-fitted socks worn over the calves to increase blood flow to the muscles. You can't miss our funky designs at races. Lots of our members wear them to be identified as part of the Run Mummy Run tribe, but they can also aid muscle recovery. Read more about compression socks in chapter one, page 45.

▶ **Core stability:** Exercises to improve your core muscles, found in your abdominals. Strengthening these muscles has many benefits from improving your posture to helping prevent stress incontinence. The plank is one exercise you can do to work your core. Read more about core stability in chapter three (page 82) and in the stress incontinence section in chapter four (page 114).

▶ **CR:** This stands for course record. Your CR might not be a personal best time, but it will be your fastest time for that particular route.

▶**Cross country running**: Another term for off-road or trail running. Cross country running could be across fields, along forest trails or round grassy park land. See more on cross country racing in chapter five.

▶**Cross training**: Cross training is exercise you do around your running to help you get fitter and stronger. Good forms of cross training that complement running are cycling, swimming, yoga and pilates.

▶**C25K**: An abbreviation for Couch To 5k, a training plan that helps beginners become runners. It uses a run-walk method and builds up week-on-week until eventually participants can run 5k (3.1 miles). Read more on C25K and see the training plan in chapter two, page 56.

▶**DNF**: Stands for did not finish. If you start a race but do not finish, for example, if you have to pull out because you feel sick or are struggling with an injury, you will be recorded in the results as DNF.

▶**DNS**: Stands for did not start. This is when you enter a race but do not take part and do not transfer your place to another runner. You may be recorded in the results as DNS.

▶**DOMS**: Stands for delayed onset muscle soreness. These are the aches and pains you get 24–36 hours after exercise. While you may feel like you have been run over by a bus, they are generally nothing to worry about and will pass in a few days. Beware though that they can make a flight of stairs feel like Mount Everest! Warming up and down, stretching, wearing compression clothing and eating protein post-run can help to prevent it. Avoid hard exercise when you are experiencing DOMS.

▶ **Drills, running:** These are moves often done over 50–100 m as part of a warm-up before an interval session or race to help you limber up and improve running form. They include running with high knees, flicking the heels to touch your bottom while running and running sideways with a wide stride. They also include doing short sprints, aka strides (see definition).

▶ **Easy run:** A run done at a comfortable pace at which you can easily hold a conversation.

▶ **Energy drinks and gels:** Products with extra carbs and sugars that can help you top up your glycogen stores when running (see the definition on carb-loading for more). You only need to top up these stores when doing a long-distance run or race. The gels can be an acquired taste as they have a sweet, sticky consistency.

▶ **Fartlek:** Possibly wins the award for most amusing term in running, but it is actually Swedish for 'speed play'. Fartlek is an informal type of speed work that can be used by runners of all levels. Rather than structured intervals of a set time or distance, you may increase your pace during a run whenever you want. This could be between objects you can see (for example, between lamp posts or 'from here to that tree', or to the top of a hill) or for varying amounts of time (e.g. running harder for one minute, jogging for a couple of minutes, then running hard again for two minutes, then jogging for two minutes, then running harder for 30 seconds). This is a fun activity when running with friends as you can take it in turns to shout the landmark to increase your pace to, or the time to keep running hard for.

▶ **Fell running:** Off-road running on mountainous terrain.

▶ **Flying feet:** A feat celebrated by RMR members that occurs when they get an action shot of themselves running with space between their feet and the ground.

▶ **Foam roller:** A hard cylindrical object that can be used to self-massage.

▶ **Frockwomble:** A female version of a cockwomble.

▶ **Gait, also gait analysis:** Your running gait refers to your form and how your foot strikes the ground when you run. Running shops carry out gait analysis so they can recommend the best trainers for your running style.

▶ **Garmin:** A brand that makes GPS watches that are popular with runners. Just like the name Hoover has become a term used to refer to a vacuum cleaner, runners will often talk about their Garmin when referring to their GPS watch.

▶**GFA:** Stands for Good for Age. The London Marathon and some other major races offer places to runners who achieve a specific time that is 'good for their age' in a qualifying marathon.

▶**GNR:** A common abbreviation for the Great North Run – the largest and most iconic half marathon in the UK. It starts in Newcastle and finishes in South Shields. RMR members voted it as their top British half marathon in our poll in chapter five, page 159.

▶**Gun time:** The time it takes you to finish a race from the moment it officially starts (i.e. when the gun goes) to when you cross the finish line. In a big race where it might take several minutes to get over the start line due to the large number of participants, your gun time can be a lot slower than your chip time.

▶**Half marathon, also half, or HM:** A race that is exactly half the distance of a marathon: 13.1 miles or 21 kilometres.

▶**Heart rate monitor:** A product used to measure the number of heartbeats per minute. Some require a band to be worn around your chest, others work via a wristwatch. Knowing your heart rate can aid your training because once you have worked out your maximum you can push yourself to it when doing hard sessions and races. Knowing your heart rate can also help you tell if you are under the weather (if so it will be higher than usual on an easy run) and help you control your effort if running when pregnant.

▶ **HIIT:** Stands for High Intensity Interval Training. This involves doing hard exercise for a short period of time, having a short rest and repeating. It can help make you fitter and burn more calories than easy exercise. You can do HIIT running sessions by running hard intervals with a short recovery e.g. 10 x 1-minute running sessions with a 30-second recovery between each.

▶ **Hitting the Wall:** A phrase synonymous with marathon running, it describes the unpleasant feeling when you run out of energy due to your glycogen stores being depleted. You will feel exhausted, heavy-legged, light-headed and may struggle to keep moving. Get your race nutrition strategy sorted to avoid this happening (see the glossary definitions on carb-loading, energy drinks and gels and the carb-loading section in chapter six, page 211).

▶ **Hydration pack:** A product favoured by ultra runners, this is a backpack with a built-in water pouch which enables you to carry a large amount of liquid on your run. They have straws attached to make accessing the water easier.

▶ **Ice bath:** Many elite athletes plunge themselves into a bath or giant bucket of icy water after a hard run or race. The theory is that it can aid recovery as exposing the body to the freezing water helps to constrict blood vessels, remove waste products and reduce swelling. It's worth noting that the jury is out on the benefit of ice baths for non-elite athletes, although many runners swear by them. If you're brave enough to try one, make it more bearable by keeping a woolly hat on and enjoying a hot cup of tea at the same time!

▶**Intervals:** Repetitions of running hard for a set period of time or a set distance with a short recovery in between e.g. 3 x 5-minute running sessions with a 90-second recovery between each or 3 x 1000 m sprint with a 400 m jog for recovery. Interval sessions can help improve your speed and fitness.

▶**IT band, also ITB:** Refers to the iliotibial band. You probably don't know what, or where, this is in your body unless you've had a problem with it, which many runners do. It is actually a band of fascia (connective tissue) that runs down your outer thigh with one end attached to your hip and the other to the outside of your knee. When it's tight it's a common cause of knee pain in runners. See the section in chapter three on 'runner's knee', page 87, for help.

▶**Jeffing:** A phrase popular with Run Mummy Run members to describe the Jeff Galloway method of run-walk training. They may 'Jeff' a marathon or 'complete a half by Jeffing'. It is a well-recognised method that claims to help runners to extend the distance they can cover with a reduced risk of injury and fatigue. See more on Jeffing in chapter two, page 53.

▶**JOGLE:** Stands for John O'Groats to Land's End. You will often see this abbreviation if someone is attempting to run from the top of Scotland to the bottom of England. You may sometimes see LE JOG if they are going the other way.

▶**Junior parkrun:** Timed 2k runs held in parks across the UK on Sunday mornings for 4–14-year-olds and their families. A fun way to get your children (and you!) into running.

▶**LiRF:** Stands for Leadership in Running Fitness. This qualification from UK Athletics means you have the knowledge and insurance to lead a run. Anyone can do the one-day course – read more about it in chapter seven, page 224.

▶**Long run:** Most runners would define a long run as an hour or more of running but technically if you only ever run for 25 minutes in the week and then 45 minutes at the weekend, then that would be your long run. Doing a run where you keep going for a longer time/distance helps improve your stamina and endurance.

▶**LSR:** Stands for Long Slow/Steady Run. Most running training plans will contain one of these runs, particularly if you are half or marathon training. The length of your

LSR will depend on the distance you are training for. The distance covered in an LSR should gradually increase over the course of your training plan and then taper towards the end. It should be done at such a pace that you still have the breath to hold a conversation comfortably.

▶ **Maranoia:** An amalgamation of the words marathon and paranoia, maranoia is experienced by some runners in the build-up to a marathon as they become nervous that they have an injury or illness that might affect their ability to take part.

▶ **Marathon:** A long-distance race measuring 26.2 miles or 42 kilometres.

▶ **Masters, also veterans:** In running terms, a master or veteran is a runner aged 35 and over (although in some races, you aren't classed as a master/vet until you are over 40). Some events have separate prizes for veteran runners and there are some vet-only competitions.

▶ **Minute-per-mile pace, also mile pace:** The speed at which you can, on average, run a mile in training. You might be asked what your mile-pace is when you join a running club so that they can put you in the correct training group for your ability.

▶ **Naked run:** Keep your clothes on! This means training without the aid of any gadgets, such as GPS watches or heart rate monitors.

▶**Negative split:** When you complete the second half of the race in a faster time than the first. For example, in a 10k you would run the second 5k in a quicker time than the first 5k. It is difficult to achieve as most people go faster in the first half when they feel fresh. However, if you can run a negative split you will be less likely to 'blow up' or 'hit the wall'.

▶**Non-cockwomble, non-CW:** The opposite of a cockwomble – they support and encourage their partners in their running endeavours.

▶**Orthotics:** Bespoke insoles that you can put in your trainers to prevent, or recover from, an injury. You shouldn't need them unless they have been recommended to you by an expert such as a physio or doctor.

▶**Paarlauf:** A training session where you run in pairs. One runs hard while the other jogs and then you switch places, doing this for a set length of time e.g. 20 minutes.

▶**Pacemaker:** Someone who helps another runner to achieve or maintain a certain pace, often used in races. The pacemaker will run at a set speed and the runner they are pacing needs to keep up with them.

▶**parkrun:** Timed 5k runs held across the UK (and in some other countries around the world) in a park at 9 a.m. every Saturday morning. It's free and anyone can take part, regardless of their ability. Read more on parkrun in chapter five, page 145.

▶**Personal best, also PB:** This is the fastest time you have run a specific distance in and an achievement that's always well-celebrated by runners.

▶**Pick-up runs, aka progression runs:** Runs where you start at an easy pace and then get faster as the miles progress.

▶**Plank, the:** An exercise to help strengthen your core, which involves balancing on your toes and forearms. See more in chapter four (page 117).

▶**Plantar fasciitis:** A common injury that runners experience in the foot. See the injury section in chapter three (page 87).

▶**Pyramid session:** An interval session where the repetitions go up in time/distance before going back down again.

▶**Race For Life:** A women-only 5k race series organised by Cancer Research UK. See more in chapter five, page 148.

▶**Race pace:** The speed at which you can run in a race. If you want to achieve a PB, your race pace should be faster than your easy and steady run pace. It should be the fastest pace you can maintain for the duration of the race.

▶**Reps:** Short for repetitions.

▶**RICE:** Stands for Rest Ice Compression Elevation. These are the first steps you are recommended to take if you have a pulled muscle or twisted ankle. Read more about it in the injury prevention section in chapter three (page 89).

▶**RMR:** The common abbreviation of Run Mummy Run. Members of the group are often referred to as RMRs (but be aware that outside of the Run Mummy Run community it can also refer to the Royal Marine Reserves!).

▶**Running belt:** Similar to a bum bag, they can be worn whilst running to carry items such as your keys and mobile. Good versions shouldn't bounce when you run.

▶**Run streak, or streaking:** Nothing to do with nudity! A run streak is where someone chooses to run every day for a period of time (this can vary) for a minimum distance (this can also vary), for instance, one mile per day for a fortnight. It can be a fun way to stay motivated but it's not recommended for too lengthy a time – we need rest and days off from running to allow our bodies to recover in order to prevent illness and injury.

▶**Senior:** In running terms, a senior is not someone elderly but someone aged 21–35.

▶**Shin splints:** A common injury runners experience that causes pain around the shin bone. Read more in the injury section in chapter three.

▶**Spikes:** A form of lightweight trainer with holes in the forefoot to screw spikes into for extra grip. This kind of shoe is mostly used when racing; track athletes will wear short spikes, while cross country runners will wear extra-long ones for better grip on muddy courses.

▶**Splits:** Not just something you can do if you're flexible! Splits for runners are the times you take to run certain intervals of distance during a run e.g. how long it takes you to run each mile of a four mile run or how much it takes you to run each 5k in a 10k race. You will run the most efficiently if you can run even splits i.e. keeping your pace the same throughout a race.

▶**Sports massage:** A very firm massage that can help alleviate muscle tension and soreness. Much more pressure tends to be applied in these than in relaxing massages so it can be painful – but it's a case of no pain, no gain!

▶**Steady run:** A run at a pace which feels comfortable but is slightly faster than your easy run pace.

▶**Strides:** This involves accelerating over a very short distance such as 50–100 m as part of a warm-up (e.g. in between a warm-up jog and the start of an interval session) or towards the end of an easy run to inject some speed and help you focus on your running form. You can then do this at the very end of a race with a sprint finish where you work all the way to the line. You could do other running drills (see definition) as well as strides as part of a warm-up before a speed session or race.

▶ **Taper, also tapering:** Towards the end of most training plans for half marathons, marathons and ultramarathons there is a period called the taper or tapering. This is a period of time when you run fewer miles and don't train as hard so that you can be fresh and well-recovered for race day. See more on tapering in chapter five, page 180.

▶ **Taping:** A method of treating some injuries. Treatment involves physios applying brightly-coloured tape to help support a certain joint or muscle group.

▶ **Tempo runs, aka threshold runs:** You will often see tempo runs pop up in your training plan. A tempo run is also sometimes known as a threshold run or a lactic-threshold run. For these you should be running at a comfortably hard pace for a set period of time/distance. You shouldn't be able to speak in sentences but you should be able to say the odd word or two. It should be about 70–80 per cent of your maximum effort. These runs are hard but you will reap the benefits.

▶ **Trail running:** This refers to off-road running. A trail run will follow trails or tracks through scenic or rural settings such as forests, hills or fields. You can buy special trainers for trail running that give you more grip on uneven surfaces and in the mud.

▶**Ultramarathon:** A race that is longer than a marathon in distance (more than 26.2 miles). There are a variety of ultra distances from 30 miles up to 100 miles or more. Some are about running for a certain distance, others for a set time, such as 24 hours. Some are multi-staged events held over a number of days.

▶**Vets, or veterans:** In running terms, this does not mean a person medically qualified to treat animals but those aged 35 plus! See more under the 'masters' definition.

▶**Virtual races:** A run where you can earn a medal (or other prize) for running a certain distance without taking part in an organised race. Read more about it in chapter five, page 192.

▶**VLM, also VMLM:** An abbreviation for the London Marathon, taking into account the sponsors Virgin Money, who have backed the event from 2010 to the time of publication.

▶**Whey protein:** Whey is a protein found in milk that can be separated from the liquid and powdered. It can be dissolved in water to create a convenient recovery drink after a hard run or race, or added to smoothies and milkshakes for extra protein.

TRAINING PLANS

Following a schedule can help you to stay motivated, enable you to stick with your training and ensure you are fully prepared for a race you've signed up for. On the following pages, we have training plans for when you're aiming for your first 10k, half marathon or marathon. If you have never run before we recommend you complete the Couch To 5k plan in chapter two (page 56) first, and then move on to these schedules.

We also have a series of 'improver' plans for 10k to marathon. These are designed to help you go faster, if that's your goal, after completing your first attempt(s) over each distance. The plans have all been devised by runner and mother-of-two, Amy Whitehead (who is also sister to the book's co-author, Lucy Waterlow). Amy is an elite runner who represented Great Britain as a junior growing up, and then went on to run for England in the marathon at the Commonwealth Games in Glasgow in 2014, juggling training with motherhood. Throughout her years as an elite runner she's been lucky enough to be advised by many expert coaches, and she's put the knowledge she has gained into these plans as well as her own expertise as a Leadership in Running Fitness graduate, and qualified post-natal fitness instructor. Amy can also write bespoke training plans for runners of all abilities. Contact her via www.runningfeat.co.uk.

RUN YOUR FIRST 10K

▶ This plan is intended to follow on from the C25K plan. If you have never run before then follow the C25K plan in chapter two (page 56) first. If you're already slightly fit and can run for 25 minutes continuously, you could start with this plan without doing the C25K.

▶ We've displayed the training on Mondays, Wednesdays and Saturdays but you can swap them for other days if it's more convenient for you but spread them out across the week so you have time to recover between sessions.

▶ Runs should be at a comfortable pace unless otherwise stated.

▶ There's a reminder to stretch and do core exercises after one run per week, but if you can fit more core exercises into your week then do so, and stretch after every run if your muscles start feeling tight. See the glossary for any training terms you don't understand (e.g. 'fartlek' or 'active recovery').

	Mon	Tue	Wed	Thur	Fri	Sat	Sun
Week 1	Run 2 miles followed by 10 min of stretching and core stability exercises	Rest	Run 2 miles	Rest or active recovery	Rest	Run 3 miles or join in your local parkrun	Rest
Week 2	Run 3 miles followed by 10 min of stretching and core stability exercises	Rest	Run 1 mile easy, run 1 mile fartlek, run 1 mile easy	Rest or active recovery	Rest	Run 3 miles or join in your local parkrun	Rest
Week 3	Run 3 miles followed by 10 min of stretching and core stability exercises	Rest	Run 1 mile easy, run 1 mile tempo pace, run 1 mile easy	Rest or active recovery	Rest	Run 3 miles or join in your local parkrun	Rest

	Mon	Tue	Wed	Thur	Fri	Sat	Sun
Week 4	Run 3 miles followed by 10 min of stretching and core stability exercises	Rest	Run 1 mile easy as a warm-up, then approx. 150 m uphill efforts x 3 with jog back recovery, then 1 mile cool-down	Rest or active recovery	Rest	Run 4 miles	Rest
Week 5	Run 3 miles followed by 10 min of stretching and core stability exercises	Rest	Run 1 mile easy, run 1 mile fartlek, run 1 mile easy	Rest or active recovery	Rest	Run 4 miles	Rest
Week 6	Run 3 miles followed by 10 min of stretching and core stability exercises	Rest	Run 1 mile easy, run 1 mile tempo pace, run 1 mile easy	Rest or active recovery	Rest	Run 5 miles	Rest

Week	Mon	Tue	Wed	Thur	Fri	Sat	Sun
7	Run 3 miles followed by 10 min of stretching and core stability exercises	Rest	Run 1 mile easy as a warm-up, then approx. 150 m uphill efforts x 4 with jog back recovery, then 1 mile cool-down	Rest or active recovery	Rest	Run 6 miles – use as dress rehearsal for race day: wear intended kit and eat breakfast at the same time you'll need to on race day (don't worry about running at race pace – this run is about gaining experience and confidence of the distance, not speed)	Rest

TRAINING PLANS

	Mon	Tue	Wed	Thur	Fri	Sat	Sun
Week 8	Run 3 miles followed by 10 min of stretching and core stability exercises	Rest	Run 3 miles	Rest or active recovery	Rest	Run 5 miles	Rest
Week 9: taper	Run 2 miles followed by 10 min of stretching and core stability exercises	Rest	Run 2 miles	Rest	Rest	Run 1 mile	Race 10k!

IMPROVERS' 10K

▶ This plan introduces interval training, extends the long run and involves running four days a week. Follow this plan if you are a more experienced runner or looking to improve your time.

▶ If you are ready to run five times a week, do 3 miles of easy running instead of resting on the Wednesdays.

▶ We have listed the training on Tuesdays, Thursdays, Saturdays and Sundays but you can mix it up if running on other days is more convenient for you. Don't do the intervals and tempo runs on consecutive days, though.

▶ Pick a route for your intervals where you can run fast safely, without having to stop to cross roads e.g. laps in a park, along a pedestrianised railway line, round a track etc. Intervals are given in time, not distance, as these are about running as fast as you can.

▶ Runs should be at a comfortable pace unless otherwise stated.

▶ There's a reminder to stretch and do core exercises after one run per week, but if you can fit more core exercises into your week then do so, and stretch after every run if your muscles start feeling tight.

	Mon	Tue	Wed	Thur	Fri	Sat	Sun
Week 1	Rest	Intervals: 1 mile jog warm-up, run hard for 3 min then walk/jog 90 seconds x 5, 1 mile jog cool-down	Rest or active recovery	Run 3 miles followed by 10 min of stretching and core stability exercises	Rest	Run 3 miles or join in your local parkrun – aim to run at a slightly faster pace than your Thursday run	Run 4 miles
Week 2	Rest	Intervals: 1 mile jog warm-up, run hard for 5 min, 4 min, 3 min, 2 min, 1 min, all with 90 sec walk/jog in between, 1 mile jog cool-down	Rest or acive recovery	Run 3 miles followed by 10 min of stretching and core stability exercises	Rest	Run 3 miles on a route with a couple of gentle uphills, push yourself a little harder on the uphills	Run 4 miles

	Mon	Tue	Wed	Thur	Fri	Sat	Sun
Week 3	Rest	Intervals: 1 mile jog warm-up, run hard for 3 min then walk/jog 90 seconds x 5, 1 mile jog cool-down	Rest or active recovery	Run 4 miles followed by 10 min of stretching and core stability exercises	Rest	Run 3 miles or join in your local parkrun – aim to run at a slightly faster pace than on your Thursday run	Run 5 miles
Week 4	Rest	Intervals: 1 mile jog warm-up, run hard for 2 min then walk/jog 1 minute x 8, 1 mile jog cool-down	Rest or active recovery	Run 4 miles followed by 10 min of stretching and core stability exercises	Rest	Run 3 miles on a route with a couple of gentle uphills, push yourself a little harder on the uphills	Run 5 miles

	Mon	Tue	Wed	Thur	Fri	Sat	Sun
Week 5	Rest	Intervals: 1 mile jog warm-up, run hard for 4 min then walk/jog 90 seconds x 4, 1 mile jog cool-down	Rest or active recovery	Run 5 miles followed by 10 min of stretching and core stability exercises	Rest	Run 1 mile easy, run 1 mile tempo, 1 mile easy	Run 6 miles
Week 6	Rest	Intervals: 1 mile jog warm-up, run hard for 2 min then walk/jog 1 min x 8, 1 mile jog cool-down	Rest or active recovery	Run 4 miles followed by 10 min of stretching and core stability exercises	Rest	Run 3 miles on a route with a couple of gentle uphills, push yourself a little harder on the uphills	Run 7 miles
Week 7	Rest	Intervals: 1 mile jog warm-up, run hard for 5 min then walk/jog 90 seconds x 3, 1 mile jog cool-down	Rest or active recovery	Run 3 miles followed by 10 min of stretching and core stability exercises	Rest	Run 3 miles or join in your local parkrun – aim to run at a slightly faster pace than on your Thursday run	Run 7 miles

	Mon	Tue	Wed	Thur	Fri	Sat	Sun
Week 8	Rest	Intervals: 1 mile jog warm-up, run hard for 5 min, 4 min, 3 min, 2 min, 1 min, all with 90 sec walk/jog in between, 1 mile jog cool-down	Rest or active recovery	Run 3 miles followed by 10 min of stretching and core stability exercises	Rest	Run 3 miles	Run 5 miles
Week 9: taper	Rest	Run 2 miles	Rest or active recovery	Run 2 miles followed by 10 min of stretching and core stability exercises	Rest	Jog 1.5 miles	Race 10k!

RUN YOUR FIRST HALF MARATHON

▶ If you have never run before, then start with the C25K plan in chapter two (page 56). Ideally, you should progress from doing the C25K to the beginners' 10k plan and then do this half marathon plan, as it's wise to build up fitness and distance gradually.

▶ We've displayed the training on Mondays, Wednesdays and Saturdays but you can swap for other days if it's more convenient for you.

▶ This plan includes a long run on a Saturday which should be done at a slow pace to build up your endurance. If you want to do parkruns, swap the Saturday runs listed to Wednesday so you still do a long, continuous run each week. Then aim to do the parkrun at a slightly faster pace than your other runs if you're doing it in place of the fartlek/hills/tempo run listed on the Wednesday.

▶ Aim to do some runs off-road so you're not always running on a hard surface.

▶ There's a reminder to stretch and do core exercises after one run per week, but if you can fit more core exercises into your week then do so, and stretch after every run if your muscles start feeling tight.

	Mon	Tue	Wed	Thur	Fri	Sat	Sun
Week 1	Run 3 miles followed by 10 min of stretching and core stability exercises	Rest	Run 4 miles	Rest or active recovery	Rest	Run 5 miles	Rest
Week 2	Run 3 miles followed by 10 min of stretching and core stability exercises	Rest	Run 4 miles	Rest or active recovery	Rest	Run 6 miles	Rest
Week 3	Run 4 miles followed by 10 min of stretching and core stability exercises	Rest	Run 4 miles	Rest or active recovery	Rest	Run 7 miles	Rest

	Mon	Tue	Wed	Thur	Fri	Sat	Sun
Week 4	Run 4 miles followed by 10 min of stretching and core stability exercises	Rest	Run 1 mile easy, 1 mile fartlek, 1 mile easy	Rest or active recovery	Rest	Run 7 miles	Rest
Week 5	Run 4 miles followed by 10 min of stretching and core stability exercises	Rest	Run 2 miles easy, run approx. 150 m uphill with jog back downhill recovery x 4, run 2 miles easy	Rest or active recovery	Rest	Run 8 miles	Rest

	Mon	Tue	Wed	Thur	Fri	Sat	Sun
Week 6	Run 3 miles followed by 10 min of stretching and core stability exercises	Rest	Run 5 miles	Rest or active recovery	Rest	Find a 10k race (race on the Sunday if you can't find a Saturday race) or run 6 miles continuously as follows: run 2 miles easy, 2 miles tempo, 2 miles easy	Rest
Week 7	Run 3 miles followed by 10 min of stretching and core stability exercises	Rest	Run 5 miles	Rest or active recovery	Rest	Run 9 miles	Rest

	Mon	Tue	Wed	Thur	Fri	Sat	Sun
Week 8	Run 4 miles followed by 10 min of stretching and core stability exercises	Rest	Run 1 mile easy, 1 mile fartlek, 1 mile easy	Rest or active recovery	Rest	Run 10 miles	Rest
Week 9	Run 4 miles followed by 10 min of stretching and core stability exercises	Rest	Run 2 miles easy, run approx. 150 m uphill with jog back downhill recovery x 5, run 2 miles easy	Rest or active recovery	Rest	Run 11 miles	Rest

	Mon	Tue	Wed	Thur	Fri	Sat	Sun
Week 10	Run 3 miles followed by 10 min of stretching and core stability exercises	Rest	Run 2 miles easy, run 2 miles tempo, run 2 miles easy	Rest or active recovery	Rest	Run 10 miles	Rest
Week 11: taper	Run 3 miles followed by 10 min of stretching and core stability exercises	Rest	Run 4 miles	Rest or active recovery	Rest	Run 8 miles	Rest
Week 12: taper	Run 3 miles followed by 10 min stretching and core stability exercises	Rest	Run 2 miles	Rest	Rest	Run 1.5 miles	Race half!

IMPROVERS' HALF MARATHON

▶ This plan introduces interval training, extends the long run and involves running four days a week. Follow this plan if you are a more experienced runner, or looking to improve your time.

▶ If you are ready to run five times a week, do an easy 3-mile run instead of resting on the Wednesdays.

▶ We have listed the training on Tuesdays, Thursdays, Saturdays and Sundays but you can mix it up if running on other days is more convenient for you. Don't do the intervals and tempo runs on consecutive days, though.

▶ Pick a route for your intervals where you can run fast safely without having to stop to cross roads, e.g. laps in a park, along a pedestrianised railway line, round a track etc. Intervals are given in time, not distance, as these are about running as fast as you can.

▶ Aim to do some of your runs off-road so you're not always on a hard surface.

▶ There's a reminder to stretch and do core exercises after one run per week, but if you can fit more core exercises into your week then do so, and stretch after every run if your muscles start feeling tight.

	Mon	Tue	Wed	Thur	Fri	Sat	Sun
Week 1	Rest	Intervals: 1 mile jog warm-up, run hard for 3 min then walk/jog 90 seconds x 5, 1 mile jog cool-down	Rest or active recovery	Run 4 miles easy followed by 10 min of stretching and core stability exercises	Rest	parkrun or run 3 miles	Run 6 miles
Week 2	Rest	Intervals: 1 mile jog warm-up, run hard for 2 min then walk/jog 1 min x 8, 1 mile cool-down	Rest or active recovery	Run 4 miles easy followed by 10 min of stretching and core stability exercises	Rest	Run 5 miles including 2 or 3 hills on the route	Run 7 miles

	Mon	Tue	Wed	Thur	Fri	Sat	Sun
Week 3	Rest	Intervals: 1 mile jog warm-up, run hard for 4 min then walk/jog 90 seconds x 4, 1 mile jog cool-down	Rest or active recovery	Run 5 miles followed by 10 min of stretching and core stability exercises	Rest	parkrun or run 3 miles – aim to do this run at your tempo pace with 1 mile warm-up and 1 mile cool-down jog before and after	Run 8 miles
Week 4	Rest	Intervals: 1 mile jog warm-up, run hard for 5 mins then walk/jog 2 mins x 4, 1 mile jog cool-down	Rest or active recovery	Run 5 miles followed by 10 min of stretching and core stability exercises	Rest	Run 5 miles pick-up i.e. start at easy pace for miles 1-2 then aim to go quicker on mile 3 (your predicted half pace) and quicker again mile 4 (your 10k pace), then easy mile 5 for a cool-down	Run 9 miles

	Mon	Tue	Wed	Thur	Fri	Sat	Sun
Week 5	Rest	Intervals: 1 mile warm-up jog, run hard for 5 min, 3 min, 1 min, all with 90 seconds jog/walk recovery in between. Walk/jog 3 min then repeat hard session, 1 mile cool-down jog	Rest or active recovery	Run 3 miles followed by 10 min of stretching and core stability exercises	Rest	Find a 10k race (race on the Sunday if there are no Saturday races you can do) or run 1 mile easy, 2 miles tempo with 800 m jog recovery x 2, 1 mile easy	Rest
Week 6	Rest	Run 4 miles followed by 10 min of stretching and core stability exercises (interval session on Thurs this week to give a longer recovery from the 10k race)	Rest or active recovery	Intervals: 1 mile warm-up jog, run hard for 2 min then walk/jog 1 min x 8, 1 mile cool-down jog	Rest	Run 5 miles including 2 to 3 hills on the route	Run 10 miles

	Mon	Tue	Wed	Thur	Fri	Sat	Sun
Week 7	Rest	Intervals: 1 mile jog warm-up, run hard for 3 min then walk/jog 90 seconds x 6, 1 mile jog cool-down	Rest or active recovery	Run 6 miles followed by 10 min of stretching and core stability exercises	Rest	parkrun or run 3 miles – aim to do this run at your tempo pace with 1 mile warm-up and 1 mile cool-down jog before and after	Run 11 miles
Week 8	Rest	Intervals: 1 mile jog warm-up, run hard for 4 min then walk/jog 90 seconds x 5, 1 mile jog cool-down	Rest or active recovery	Run 6 miles followed by 10 min of stretching and core stability exercises	Rest	Run 5 miles off-road including 2 or 3 hills on the route	Run 12 miles

	Mon	Tue	Wed	Thur	Fri	Sat	Sun
Week 9	Rest	Intervals: 1 mile jog warm-up, run hard for 5 min then walk/jog 2 min x 4, 1 mile jog cool-down	Rest or active recovery	Run 5 miles followed by 10 min of stretching and core stability exercises	Rest	parkrun or run 3 miles – aim to do this run at your tempo pace with 1 mile warm up and 1 mile cool down jog before and after	Run 12 miles
Week 10	Rest	Intervals: 1 mile jog warm-up, run hard for 3 min then walk/jog 90 seconds x 6, 1 mile jog cool-down	Rest or active recovery	Run 4 miles followed by 10 min of stretching and core stability exercises	Rest	Run 1 mile easy, 2 miles tempo with 800 m jog recovery x 2, 1 mile easy	Run 11 miles

TRAINING PLANS

	Mon	Tue	Wed	Thur	Fri	Sat	Sun
Week 11: taper	Rest	Intervals: 1 mile jog warm-up, run hard for 1 min then walk/jog for 1 min x 10, 1 mile jog cool-down	Rest or active recovery	Run 4 miles followed by 10 min of stretching and core stability exercises	Rest	Run 4 miles	Run 8 miles
Week 12: taper!	Rest	Run 3 miles	Rest or active recovery	Run 2 miles followed by 10 min of stretching and core stability exercises	Rest	Jog 1.5 miles	Race half!

RUN YOUR FIRST MARATHON

▶ If you have never run before, then start with the C25K plan in chapter two (page 56). Ideally, you should progress from doing the C25K to the beginners' 10k plan, to the beginners' half marathon plan, as it's wise to build up fitness and distance gradually.

▶ If you are going straight from C25K to this plan, give yourself 20 weeks to train instead of the 15 below and follow weeks one to five of the Run Your First Half marathon plan first.

▶ We've displayed the training on Tuesdays, Thursdays, Saturdays and Sundays but you can swap for other days if it's more convenient for you. If you can only fit in running three times a week, drop the Saturday run. Also, drop the Saturday run if you find you are getting too fatigued because, as the plan progresses, the Sunday run gets longer. It's much more important that you complete the long Sunday run so if you feel you need to be fresher for it, rest on the Saturday.

▶ If you want to join in a parkrun for your Saturday run then don't run hard because you don't want to be tired for your long Sunday run. Treat the parkruns as an opportunity to do your run with company and not as a race*.

▶ Don't run too fast on the long Sunday run; they are about gaining endurance and confidence and not about speed.

▶ Tempo runs should be done at a slightly faster pace than usual but not flat out. These are to add some variety to your training and help improve fitness.

▶ Aim to do some of your runs off-road so you're not always running on a hard surface.

▶ There's a reminder to stretch and do core exercises after one run per week, but if you can fit more core exercises into your week then do so, and stretch after every run if your muscles start feeling tight.

	Mon	Tue	Wed	Thur	Fri	Sat	Sun
Week 1	Rest	Run 3 miles	Rest or active recovery	Run 4 miles followed by 10 min of stretching and core stability exercises	Rest	Run 3 miles or join in your local parkrun*	Run 10 miles
Week 2	Rest	Run 3 miles	Rest or active recovery	Run 4 miles followed by 10 min of stretching and core stability exercises	Rest	Run 3 miles or join in your local parkrun*	Run 10 miles
Week 3	Rest	Run 1 mile easy, 1 mile tempo, 1 mile easy	Rest or active recovery	Run 4 miles followed by 10 min of stretching and core stability exercises	Rest	Run 3 miles or join in your local parkrun*	Run 12 miles
Week 4	Rest	Run 1 mile easy, 1 mile fartlek, 1 mile easy	Rest or active recovery	Run 5 miles followed by 10 min of stretching and core stability exercises	Rest	Run 3 miles or join in your local parkrun*	Run 12 miles

	Mon	Tue	Wed	Thur	Fri	Sat	Sun
Week 5	Rest	Run 1 mile easy, 1 mile tempo, 1 mile easy	Rest or active recovery	Run 5 miles followed by 10 min of stretching and core stability exercises	Rest	Run 3 miles or join in your local parkrun*	Run 14 miles
Week 6	Rest	Run 1 mile easy, run 150 m uphill with jog back recovery x 5, run 1 mile easy	Rest or active recovery	Run 5 miles followed by 10 min of stretching and core stability exercises	Rest	Run 3 miles or join in your local parkrun*	Run 14 miles
Week 7	Rest	Run 1 mile easy, run mile tempo, run 1 mile easy	Rest or active recovery	Run 6 miles followed by 10 min of stretching and core stability exercises	Rest	Run 3 miles or join in your local parkrun*	Run 16 miles

RUN MUMMY RUN

	Mon	Tue	Wed	Thur	Fri	Sat	Sun
Week 8	Rest	Run 1 mile easy, run 1 fartlek, run 1 mile easy	Rest or active recovery	Run 6 miles followed by 10 min of stretching and core stability exercises	Rest	Run 3 miles or join in your local parkrun*	Run 18 miles
Week 9	Rest	Run 1 mile easy, run 150 m uphill with jog back recovery x 5, run 1 mile easy	Rest or active recovery	Run 6 miles followed by 10 min of stretching and core stability exercises	Rest	Run 3 miles or join in your local parkrun*	Run 15 miles (mini-taper ahead of half marathon next week)
Week 10	Rest	Run 3 miles	Rest or active recovery	Run 4 miles followed by 10 min of stretching and core stability exercises	Rest	Run 2 miles	Race a half marathon
Week 11	Rest	Run 3 miles	Rest or active recovery	Run 5 miles followed by 10 min of stretching and core stability exercises	Rest	Run 3 miles or join in your local parkrun*	Run 18 miles

	Mon	Tue	Wed	Thur	Fri	Sat	Sun
Week 12	Rest	Run 1 mile easy, run mile tempo, run 1 mile easy	Rest or active recovery	Run 5 miles followed by 10 min of stretching and core stability exercises	Rest	Run 3 miles or join in your local parkrun*	Run 20 miles
Week 13: taper	Rest	Run 3 miles	Rest or active recovery	Run 4 miles followed by 10 min of stretching and core stability exercises	Rest	Run 2 miles	Run 15 miles
Week 14: taper	Rest	Run 3 miles	Rest or active recovery	Run 3 miles followed by 10 min of stretching and core stability exercises	Rest	Run 2 miles	Run 8 miles
Week 15: taper	Rest	Run 2 miles	Rest	Run 1 mile	Rest	Run 1 mile easy	Race marathon!

IMPROVERS' MARATHON

▶This plan introduces interval training, extends the long run and involves running four days a week. Follow this plan if you are a more experienced runner looking to run your first marathon after doing a few halfs, or looking to improve your marathon time.

▶We have listed the training on Tuesdays, Thursdays, Saturdays and Sundays but you can mix it up if running on other days is more convenient for you. Don't do the intervals and pick-up/marathon pace runs on consecutive days, though.

▶The Sunday run should be at an easy pace to build up your endurance – save going faster for the interval sessions and marathon-paced runs listed.

▶There's a reminder to stretch and do core exercises after one run per week, but if you can fit more core exercises into your week then do so, and stretch after every run if your muscles start feeling tight.

▶Aim to do some runs off-road so you're not always running on a hard surface.

	Mon	Tue	Wed	Thur	Fri	Sat	Sun
Week 1	Rest	Intervals: jog 1 mile warm-up, run hard for 3 min then walk/jog 1 min x 6, jog 1 mile cool-down	Rest or active recovery	Run 5 miles, followed by 10 min of stretching and core stability exercises	Rest	Run 3 miles or join in your local parkrun at a slightly faster pace than your Thursday run	Run 10 miles
Week 2	Rest	Intervals: jog 1 mile warm-up, run hard for 4 min, walk/jog 90 sec x 4, jog 1 mile cool-down	Rest or active recovery	Run 5 miles, followed by 10 min of stretching and core stability exercises	Rest	Run 5 miles including 2 to 3 hills on the route	Run 10 miles
Week 3	Rest	Intervals: jog 1 mile warm-up, run hard for 5 min, walk/jog 90 sec x 4, jog 1 mile cool-down	Rest or active recovery	Run 6 miles, followed by 10 min of stretching and core stability exercises	Rest	Run 1 mile easy, 3 miles at predicted marathon pace (or parkrun at marathon pace), 1 mile easy	Run 12 miles

Week 4	Mon	Tue	Wed	Thur	Fri	Sat	Sun
	Rest	Intervals: jog 1 mile warm-up, run hard for 3 min, walk/jog 2 min x 6, jog 1 mile cool-down	Rest or active recovery	Run 6 miles, followed by 10 min of stretching and core stability exercises	Rest	Run 5 miles 'pick-up', i.e. start at easy pace for miles 1 and 2 then aim to go quicker on mile 3 (predicted marathon pace) and quicker again mile 4 (your half marathon pace), then run mile 5 easy for a cool-down	Run 14 miles

	Mon	Tue	Wed	Thur	Fri	Sat	Sun
Week 5	Rest	Intervals: jog 1 mile warm-up, run hard for 2 min, walk/jog 1 min x 8, jog 1 mile cool-down	Rest or active recovery	Run 5 miles, followed by 10 min of stretching and core stability exercises	Rest	Run 2 miles	Race 10K (if you can't find a 10K race on this weekend, do parkrun on Sat instead at race pace with a mile easy before and 2 miles easy after)
Week 6	Rest	Run 4 miles	Rest or active recovery	Run 6 miles, followed by 10 min of stretching and core stability exercises	Rest	Run 5 miles including 2 to 3 hills on the route	Run 16 miles
Week 7	Rest	Intervals: jog 1 mile warm-up, run hard for 5 min, rest for 90 sec x 4, jog 1 mile cool-down	Rest or active recovery	Run 7 miles, followed by 10 min of stretching and core stability exercises	Rest	Run 1 mile easy, run 3 miles at predicted marathon pace (or parkrun at marathon pace), run 1 mile easy	Run 16 miles

	Mon	Tue	Wed	Thur	Fri	Sat	Sun
Week 8	Rest	Intervals: 1 mile warm-up jog, run hard for 5 min, 3 min, 1 min, all with 90 seconds jog/walk recovery in between. Walk/jog 3 min then repeat, 1 mile cool-down	Rest or active recovery	Run 7 miles, followed by 10 min of stretching and core stability exercises	Rest	Run 5 miles 'pick-up', i.e. start at easy pace for miles 1 and 2 then aim to go quicker on mile 3 (predicted marathon pace) and quicker again mile 4 (your half marathon pace), then run mile 5 easy for a cool-down	Run 18 miles

	Mon	Tue	Wed	Thur	Fri	Sat	Sun
Week 9	Rest	Intervals: jog 1 mile warm-up, run hard for 3 min, walk/jog 2 min x 6, jog 1 mile cool-down	Rest or active recovery	Run 8 miles, followed by 10 min of stretching and core stability exercises	Rest	Run 5 miles including 2 to 3 hills on the route	Run 15 miles (mini taper ahead of half marathon)
Week 10	Rest	Intervals: jog 1 mile warm-up, run hard for 2 min, walk/jog 1 min x 8, jog 1 mile cool-down	Rest or active recovery	Run 6 miles, followed by 10 min of stretching and core stability exercises	Rest	Run 2 miles	Race a half marathon

	Mon	Tue	Wed	Thur	Fri	Sat	Sun
Week 11	Rest	Run 4 miles	Rest or active recovery	Run 7 miles, followed by 10 min of stretching and core stability exercises	Rest	Run 5 miles 'pick-up', i.e. start at easy pace for miles 1 and 2 then aim to go quicker on mile 3 (predicted marathon pace) and quicker again mile 4 (your half marathon pace), then run mile 5 easy for a cool-down	Run 20 miles
Week 12	Rest	Intervals: Jog 1 mile warm-up, run hard for 6 min, walk/jog 2 min x 3, jog 1 mile cool-down	Rest or active recovery	Run 8 miles, followed by 10 min of stretching and core stability exercises	Rest	Run 1 mile easy, run 3 miles at predicted marathon pace (or parkrun at marathon pace), run 1 mile easy	Run 20 miles

	Mon	Tue	Wed	Thur	Fri	Sat	Sun
Week 13: taper	Rest	Intervals: Jog 1 mile warm-up, run hard for 3 mins, walk/jog 1 min x 5, jog 1 mile cool-down	Rest or active recovery	Run 5 miles, followed by 10 min of stretching and core stability exercises	Rest	Run 5 miles including 2 to 3 hills on the route	Run 15 miles
Week 14: taper	Rest	Intervals: jog 1 mile warm-up, run hard for 1 min, walk/jog 1 min x 10, jog 1 mile cool-down	Rest or active recovery	Run 4 miles, followed by 10 min of stretching and core stability exercises	Rest	Run 1 mile easy, 2 miles at marathon pace, 1 mile easy	Run 8 miles
Week 15: taper	Rest	Run 3 miles	Rest	Run 2 miles	Rest	Run 1 mile easy	Race marathon!

HOW TO STAY PART OF THE RMR COMMUNITY

You've nearly reached the end of this book, but that doesn't mean it's the end of your journey with RMR! If you're not already a member of our Facebook group then do send a request to join so you can stay part of our friendly community. In the group you will find lots more advice and tips on running and you can post any running-related questions you have – we'd love to hear from you!

If you are already a member, then we hope you will continue to enjoy being part of the RMR tribe, and don't forget that there are lots of ways to get involved offline as well as online. Sign up for our newsletter by visiting www. runmummyrun.co.uk and you'll be kept fully up-to-date on our race reviews, meet-ups including sociable group runs, and how to get hold of our colourful RMR kit.

From a small group of women, RMR has grown to tens of thousands of members and, as we expand, we continue to pride ourselves on the closeness of our community. Just as the group was originally set up to enable women to meet up and run, we want to continue to help connect female runners with one another and nurture friendships. If you want to try to find runners near you to meet up with then post on the Facebook group to find those close by, or ask for local club recommendations. Via our Facebook group, members can also request to access our RMR Area Groups for different regions of the UK. This allows members to find other running buddies near them so they can meet up for training (or just for a cuppa!).

For big races around the UK, we set up online event groups so participants can share the build-up to the race together and support one another in their training. They can then arrange to meet up on the day or to run together if they are of a similar pace. A race can be a lot more fun when it's an experience shared with others. It all helps to quell any pre-race nerves and allows friendships to flourish.

We strongly believe that women empower other women, so come and join our tribe and immerse yourself in a world of positivity with those who are also passionate about running. Here are just some of the reasons why our members love being part of RMR and recommend you come and join the fun.

'Without the support of RMR I wouldn't have got through some of the hardest points in my life so far. Without this community there is no way I would've ever considered taking on some of the challenges I have, such as ultramarathons and obstacle course races. These ladies are always here with positive support and encouragement. RMR is my running family and I have made some amazing, lifelong friends.'

Lisa Mia Edwards

'No matter what time of day or night there's always someone willing to offer support and advice. It's a place where you can be truly honest and get good honest advice in return.'

Jules Reklaw

'RMR members are so supportive. They get how it feels to have a good run and how frustrating having an injury is, and there's always someone to offer advice and just that little nudge of encouragement.'

Emma Moomin Clifford

'Being part of RMR has shown me that running isn't just a sport for the super-elite but a sport for everyone. Seeing women of all ages, shapes and sizes putting their trainers on and getting out the door inspires me to do it too. And now I love running!'

Victoria Hall

'Being part of RMR gives me inspiration and motivation when I'm having down days and celebrates all different shapes and sizes and levels of fitness and pace. There are no discriminations here, it's a safe place to talk about running and get support. It also makes me laugh and makes me feel part of something great!'

Helen Chaldecott

'It's a caring and sharing community. It's great for lots of running-related chats with women who like to run, to name just a few topics – cockwombles (good and bad), chafing, underwear, toilet habits, women's issues, rants, support, worries, inspiration and motivation.'

Rach Hatters

'RMR is a perfect group for supporting new runners. I'm a beginner but still get lots of friendly comments when I post about runs which would be short or slow to others. I love seeing the inspiration of other RMRs completing marathons.'

Beth Lambert-Matthews

'Since joining I have had the confidence to go further in miles and be proud of my achievements. I'm finding myself wanting to do more runs, and I love getting, as well as giving, support. To me this group is like an extended family. There is always someone who has been there, done that.'

Rachel Shepherd

'I've never believed in me, but RMR does! I've gone from (as my mum refers to me) "the least likely person to run, ever" to being part of a fabulous group! I now run knowing I have thousands of women cheering me on!'

Claire Daniels

'Being part of RMR has meant signing up for more races than I knew existed, and knowing that, whatever race I sign up for, there will be another RMR member there with me or somebody spectating that will shout "RMR!" just when I need the boost. In this group you will meet and make lifelong running buddies. The wealth of knowledge and wisdom, help and advice available 24/7 from everyone on RMR is amazing.'

Michelle Poultney

'When starting out on your own running journey, being part of RMR gives you support from the start. Your Facebook friends might get "fed up" with your running posts – all you want to do is share your personal achievements – but you can do that on RMR and get the confidence boost you need. It's a fabulous platform for advice, which in turn you can pass on to others who are starting their running journey.'

Trinkerry White

'This group has been motivational and inspirational. Every day I see women of all ages, shapes, sizes and backgrounds running all distances and paces. It has shown me that I can do it too. On days when I want to give up or don't want to go running, I see all the other women sharing their successes and it makes me want a piece of it. It's also opened my eyes to virtual races, which I had never done before, and I find virtual races really motivating.'

Victoria Jones

'Seeing people talk about going running and enjoying it – as well as the sheer amount of posts that pop up on my Facebook feed – makes me want to go out running more. Often it helps keep you motivated and sometimes gives you that extra little push out of the door!'

Lisa Edwards

'RMR has given me back my self-confidence and I have the best new friends!'

Bunty Rance

'Being a part of RMR to me is the feeling of solidarity –
we are all in this together, regardless of how long we have
been running. It doesn't matter how far or how fast you
can run, we all support each other and celebrate each
other's achievements. Everyone is always so helpful too if
you are having a "down" period about running. There is
no nastiness – it's like we are one big, virtual family who
happen to share a love of running.'

Katie Griffiths

'It gives me a virtual kick up the bum to go out for a
run on those days I don't want to... I have a read
through the page and get myself changed and out the
door! These ladies understand!'

Sarah King

'It provides the motivation to try a little bit harder and
go a little further as well as the recognition that we
need to be gentle on ourselves and celebrate the smallest
achievements.'

Lorna Coy

'Without RMR I wouldn't still be running – simples! I have made some amazing friends whose paths I wouldn't have crossed without this amazing group. And buying some pretty funky kit too is a bonus.'

Kelly Reeves

'Since joining this group I've gained a lot more confidence in running. It's starting to feel more natural, as I know lots of people have bad runs too – it's not just me. The sense of community, love, and spirit is fantastic. It's given me a real boost, and a sense of "I can do this".'

Katie Louise Burton

'Usually when someone says they're a runner a certain stereotype comes to mind, but RMR shows that you can be a woman of any age, shape or race. The support is phenomenal, we all have good days and bad days and there's not a nasty word in sight.'

Amanda Howard

'I was introduced to RMR by my sister-in-law and I'm eternally grateful! What an inspirational group of ladies. RMRs have certainly helped me on my journey. You make me laugh and cry, and you give me that motivation to get out there.'

Sally Rollinson-Blundell

'What makes me stay in RMR? It's because I am never alone! I have posted on the group in the middle of the night while doing an ultra and got a response. I have been on top of big hill and got a response. I have been in bed needing to run and got a response. Who needs therapy when you have running shoes and RMR in your life?'

Belinda Bryant

Join our Facebook group: **www.facebook.com/ groups/runmummyrun/**

Visit our website for news and kit and to sign up for our newsletter: **www.runmummyrun.co.uk**

Follow us on Twitter **@run_mummy_run**, on Instagram **@run_mummy_run_news** and on Pinterest: **www.pinterest.com/runmummyrunRMR**

RMR MISSION STATEMENT

Run Mummy Run is the leading online running network for female runners of its kind. We've brought together tens of thousands of women with a passion for running, and built a strong community that we're incredibly proud of.

For us, as a community and as a brand, kindness is everything. We want women to be kind to themselves and follow their dreams and passions. We want women to be kind to each other, encouraging, supporting and motivating with every step. We actively promote kindness, friendship, love, support, equality and unity as our core values.

We encourage each and every member to pay it forward, and we have witnessed some amazing acts of generosity. We have built a strong, loyal team, who work tirelessly to ensure that the Run Mummy Run community stays true to our valued ethos of kindness, a place where all opinions are welcome but all must be respected.

Our aim is to encourage, support and inspire all women to take up running and enjoy their journey. We want to be there to help women through the tough times, share their milestones and celebrate their achievements. We want to provide a safe, secure environment for everyone to talk openly and honestly about every aspect of running, and a place where people know that they'll be met with kindness, respect and love. We watch as strong friendships grow both online and in real-life, and we see lives change for the better through a shared interest.

We're passionate about encouraging the next generation to be active, and we believe that by supporting women in their running journeys they become role-models for their children, inspiring them and promoting self-belief.

We carry our passion through everything we do. We take our time thoroughly researching every product that we sell in our shop – we want to provide high-quality running kit that is designed for female runners, by female runners. We want our runners to feel proud to wear our name and identify themselves as part of the Run Mummy Run tribe.

Run Mummy Run (www.runmummyrun.co.uk): The online community that values kindness, encourages self-belief, inspires dreams and supports women at every step of their running journey.

ACKNOWLEDGEMENTS

Firstly, our thanks to Summersdale for publishing this book and helping RMR to reach even more women and to inspire, support and help them get active.

We are grateful to all the RMR members who have shared their tips and experiences in the book. There are too many wonderful women to list here but thank you all for your contributions, from your reasons to run to voting for your favourite races. We'd also like to thank the members who shared their stories in more detail – Michelle Foreman, Nicky Lopez, Isobel Monaghan, Hannah Hiscock, Kate Glascott and Bianca Pridham. We said at the start that the RMR group is so amazing because of the people in it, and the many members who have contributed to this book illustrate that.

We'd also like to thank the experts who have given their time and knowledge to enhance the information provided – thank you Wendy Rumble (www.runningbuggies.com) for your tips on training with a running buggy, Debbie

Watts (www.molevalleyfitness.co.uk) for recommending strengthening exercises, Jenni Russell (www.jennirussell.com) for advice on strengthening the pelvic floor muscles and Russ Best (www.simplyrussbest.me) for your input on the best nutrition for runners.

For the training plans featured, thank you Public Health England for allowing us to reproduce your Couch To 5K plan, which is very popular with our members. The One You Couch to 5K app has been designed to get you off the couch and running in just nine weeks. Grab your trainers, download the app and follow the step-by-step instructions. You can download the app from the app store from any smart phone. Read more at www.nhs.uk/oneyou/apps.

Thanks also to Amy Whitehead (www.runningfeat.co.uk) for the other training plans featured, and to RMR's Fiona Wright for helping to compile the glossary.

Finally, thank you for reading! We hope the book inspires you to start, or carry on, running and that it has given you lots of useful advice to help you along the way. If you're reading because you're already part of the RMR community, then thank you for all your support so far. If this book has introduced you to us, then do stay involved by joining our Facebook group, following our social media channels and signing up for our newsletter via our website (see page 309). Run Mummy Run is a place to find friendships, gain in confidence and enjoy all the good that running brings. We hope to meet you soon!

LEANNE'S THANKS

There have been so many people on my Run Mummy Run journey that deserve a thank you, and so many supportive friends and family, that I wish I could mention you all, but I will do that in person. For the book I have these people to thank:

To my team – the ladies behind the scenes who volunteer their days, evenings and weekends to ensure the community runs smoothly and safely, with our members fully supported and happy. The time, loyalty and dedication you give to Run Mummy Run is incredible and you are not only the backbone of our community but my absolute rocks. You have never let me or the members down, and I love working alongside you all on this fun adventure – I could not ask for a better team.

To my dearest friend Jane, who's been my buddy since I was three. There isn't a time in our 37 years of friendship that you haven't been there for me – you are one of my biggest supporters in everything I do including Run Mummy Run, and I am so proud to call you my friend. Promise me you will keep laughing at me always!

To my parents who have always been there for me no matter what, who gave me a fun and stable upbringing and supported me throughout – my dad, who showed me the excitement of having a dream and trying to catch it, and my mum, my friend, whom I love spending time with and talking to; I just wish there were more moments like that. Thank you both for everything, I love you so much.

To the most important people in my world, my husband Guy and my little treasures Samuel and Ollie. You have sacrificed a lot to support me in building Run Mummy Run. I know there are times when I drive you all crazy with all the plans, activities, late nights and weekend work, but you can be safe in the knowledge that this wife-and-mum is the happiest she's ever been in her life. Thank you for letting me live out my dream and for sharing all the highs and lows with me. I'm so lucky to have you by my side.

And finally, my last thank you is to our Run Mummy Run members, a community of women that have changed my life. Five years ago I was a very different person – quiet, nervous, worried about what people thought of me. Fast forward and I cannot believe where I am. You have given me the kind of confidence and happiness I never thought I would find. I have made new friendships that will last a lifetime and laughed more than I ever thought possible. I am complete in every part of my life and that is down to you, my truly wonderful ladies.

Follow Leanne on Instagram @run_mummy_run_rmr.

LUCY'S THANKS

First of all I have to say a massive thank you to Leanne for trusting me with your 'baby' in allowing me to help you create a book celebrating Run Mummy Run. It has been a pleasure to immerse myself in the community you have built and get to know you and many of the other lovely members.

My own running journey started thanks to my amazing family, with my marathon-mad dad, Roy, and ever supportive mum, Sandy, encouraging me to run as a child. They made sport an everyday part of life for me and my sister. I'm so grateful as running has enriched my life in many ways, from the friendships I have made (too many to name here!), to the places I have seen, and the races that have pushed me to be the best I can be. Along with my parents, my sister Amy has always been an inspiration and great support. She's shown me that with hard work and dedication, along with a happy disposition, you can achieve your dreams – in her case, running for her country (alongside being a wonderful mum to Holly and Autumn) and in mine, running to the best of my ability and becoming a published author. I'm also grateful to her for contributing the training plans for this book which we hope will help many women to get fitter (and faster, if they wish). It's also thanks to running that I met my wonderful husband Ed via our fab local club St Albans Striders. I have been introduced to the term 'cockwomble' since joining RMR and I'm glad to say he's definitely not one of them and always supports me no matter what.

Follow Lucy on Twitter @lucyrunningfeat and Instagram @runningfeat.

REFERENCES

▶**Calories burned running:** www.womensrunning.
competitor.com/2015/04/health-wellness/weight-loss/
how-many-calories-does-running-burn_37198

www.runnersworld.com/weight-loss/how-many-
calories-are-you-really-burning

▶**Sport England survey:** www.sportengland.org/news-
and-features/news/2014/october/31/this-girl-can/

▶**Benefits for runners who wear compression garments:**
www.ncbi.nlm.nih.gov/pubmed/2710 6555

▶**Run-walk study:** www.jsams.org/article/S1440-2440%2
814%2900218-7/abstract

▶**Exercise and pregnancy:** www.rcm.org.uk/news-views-
and-analysis/news/study-highlights-benefits-of-exercising-
while-pregnant

www.nhs.uk/conditions/pregnancy-and-baby/pages/
pregnancy-exercise.aspx

▶**Knee pain study:** www.runnersworld.com/runners-knee

▶ **Exercise and the menopause studies:** www.medicaldaily. com/menopausal-women-can-reap-exercise-benefits-reduce-risk-hot-flashes-and-night-401032
www.irishtimes.com/life-and-style/health-family/yes-menopause-has-an-upside-you-could-get-fitter-1.3030664

▶ **Exercise and breastfeeding:** www.breastfeeding.asn.au/ bfinfo/exercise-and-breastfeeding

▶ **Children and exercise:** www.who.int/dietphysical activity/factsheet_young_people/en/

▶ **NHS Eatwell guide:** www.nhs.uk/Livewell/Goodfood/ Documents/The-Eatwell-Guide-2016.pdf

▶ **Beetroot for improved performance:** www.telegraph. co.uk/news/health/news/9226576/Eating-beetroot-may-improve-running-speed-research.html

▶ **Nuts for healthy diet:** www.medicalnewstoday.com/ articles/269206.php

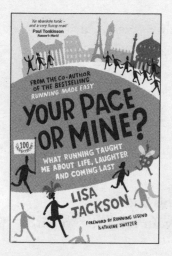

YOUR PACE OR MINE?

Lisa Jackson

ISBN: 978 1 84953 827 5

£9.99

Lisa Jackson is a surprising cheerleader for the joys of running. Formerly a committed fitness-phobe, she became a marathon runner at 31, and ran her first 56-mile ultramarathon aged 41. And unlike many runners, Lisa's not afraid to finish last – in fact, she's done so in 20 of the 90-plus marathons she's completed so far.

But this isn't just Lisa's story, it's also that of the extraordinary people she's met along the way – tutu-clad fun-runners, octogenarians and 250-mile ultrarunners – whose tales of loss and laughter are sure to inspire you just as much as they've inspired her. This book is for anyone who longs to experience the sense of connection and achievement that running has to offer, whether a nervous novice or a seasoned marathoner dreaming of doing an ultra. An account of the triumph of tenacity over a lack of talent, *Your Pace or Mine?* is proof that running really isn't about the time you do, but the time you have!

Have you enjoyed this book?
If so, why not write a review on your favourite website?

If you're interested in finding out more about our books,
find us on Facebook at **Summersdale Publishers** and
follow us on Twitter at **@Summersdale**.

Thanks very much for buying this Summersdale book.

www.summersdale.com